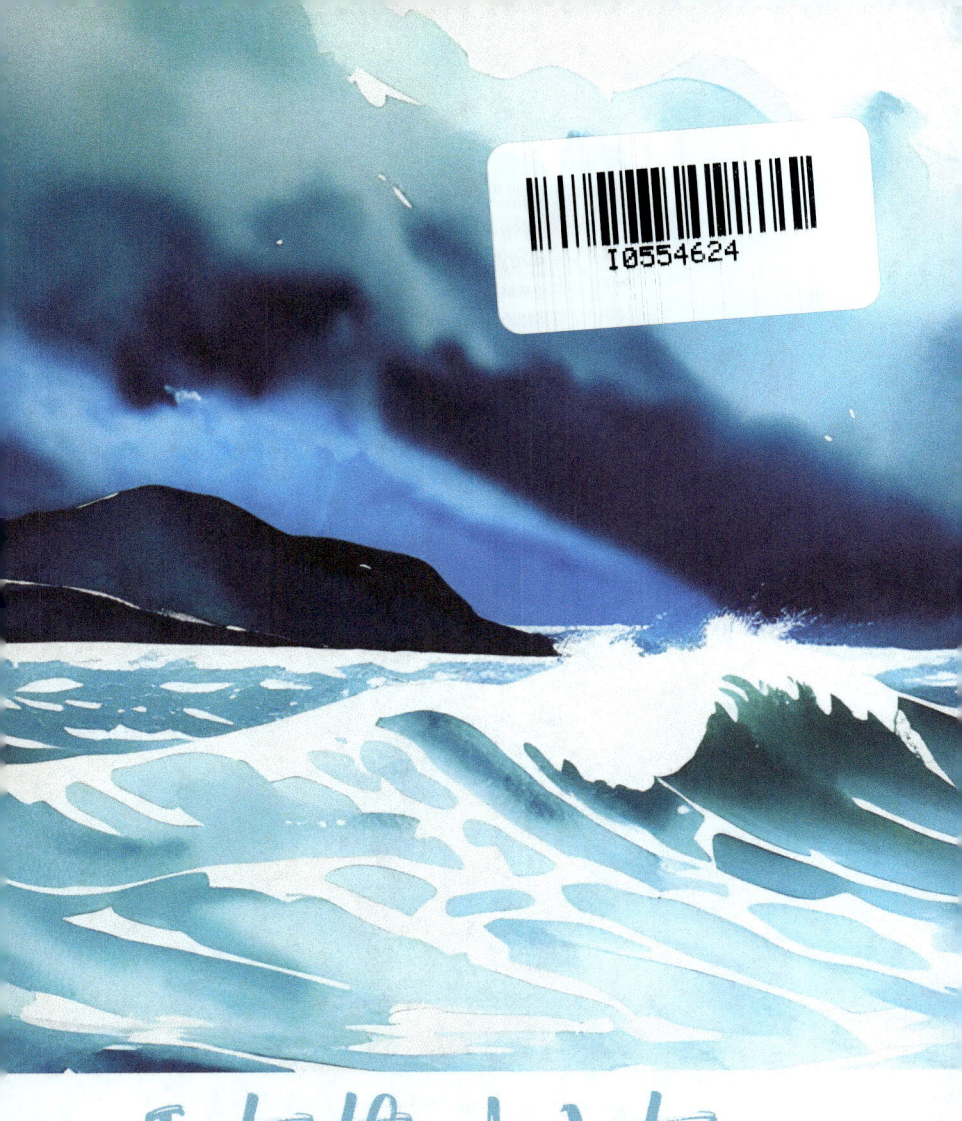

Into the Water

Wading Through Grief

A Devotional

by Marya Patrice Sherron

Into the Water
Wading Through Grief
A Devotional

All scriptures are in the New International Version.

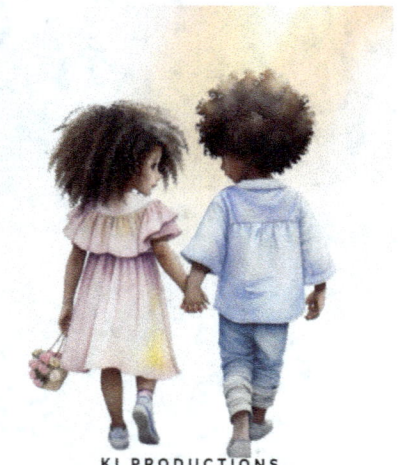

KI PRODUCTIONS
Where every story matters

Dedication

I dedicate this book to the many who walked alongside me through the various spaces and places my heart wandered. Sweet voices, often communicated through a comment on social media, called me out of the dark caves and crevices of my mind to offer hope. I am particularly grateful for those that allowed me to grieve without time constraints. One can grow weary while walking with someone who is mourning — if my circle grew tired, they never let me know.

I dedicate this to my friends and loved ones who suffered loss of their own yet demonstrated great love and resilience in the midst of their pain. Perhaps unintentional, but you offered me hope.

Finally, I dedicate this book to my parents who have endured the unimaginable. My heart has a particular ache for them — as a mother of two amazing sons, I can imagine no greater grief than that of burying a child. Abruptly. Publicly. Still, they persevere and try to find beauty in the echoes, fragrances, and love embedded in our memories. My mother did not take a moment to ponder when I invited her to contribute to this project. For the first time, she has put her feelings and thoughts on the page. I recognize how difficult it must have been and I honor her for saying yes.

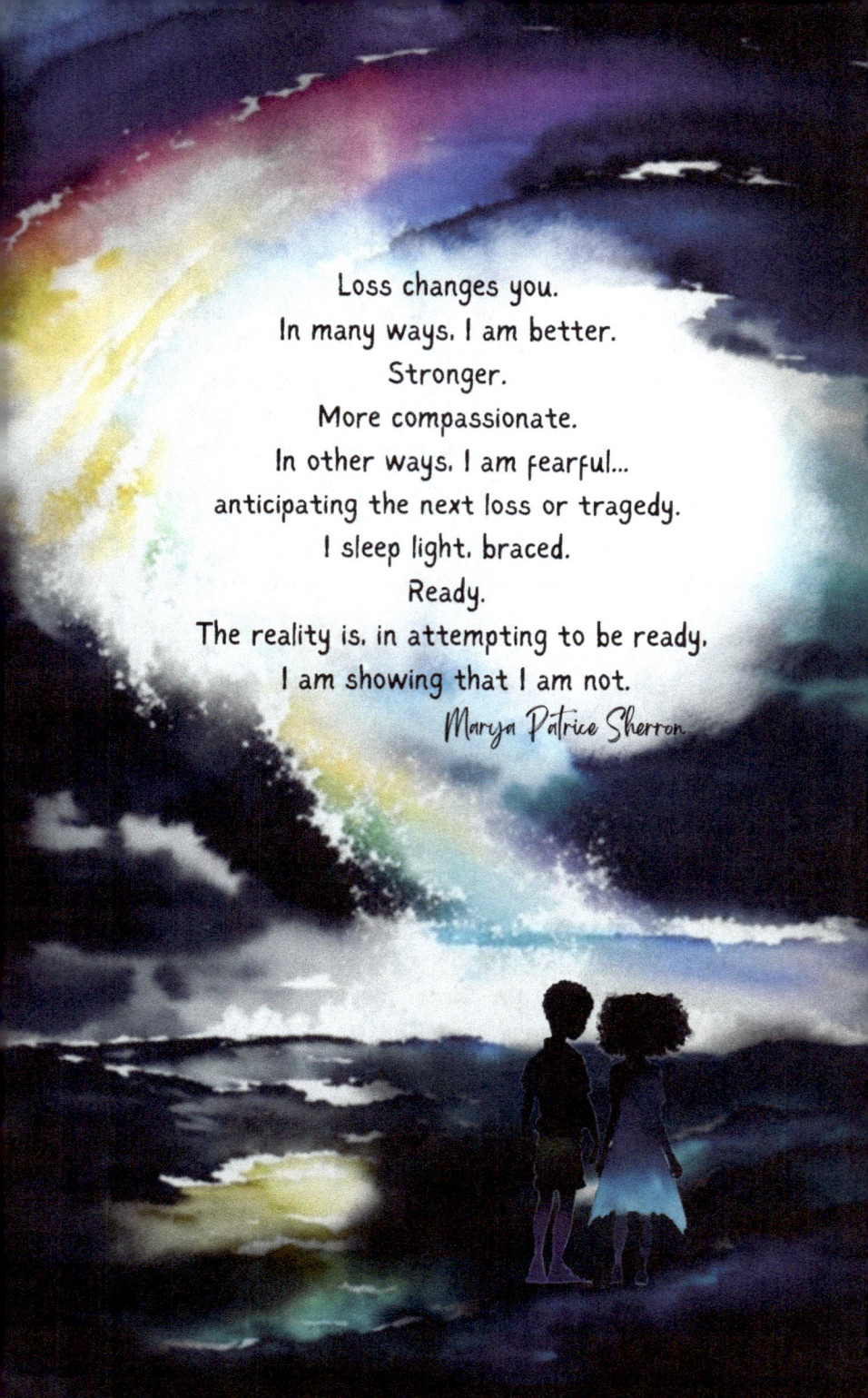

Loss changes you.
In many ways, I am better.
Stronger.
More compassionate.
In other ways, I am fearful...
anticipating the next loss or tragedy.
I sleep light, braced.
Ready.
The reality is, in attempting to be ready,
I am showing that I am not.

Marya Patrice Sherron

This belongs to

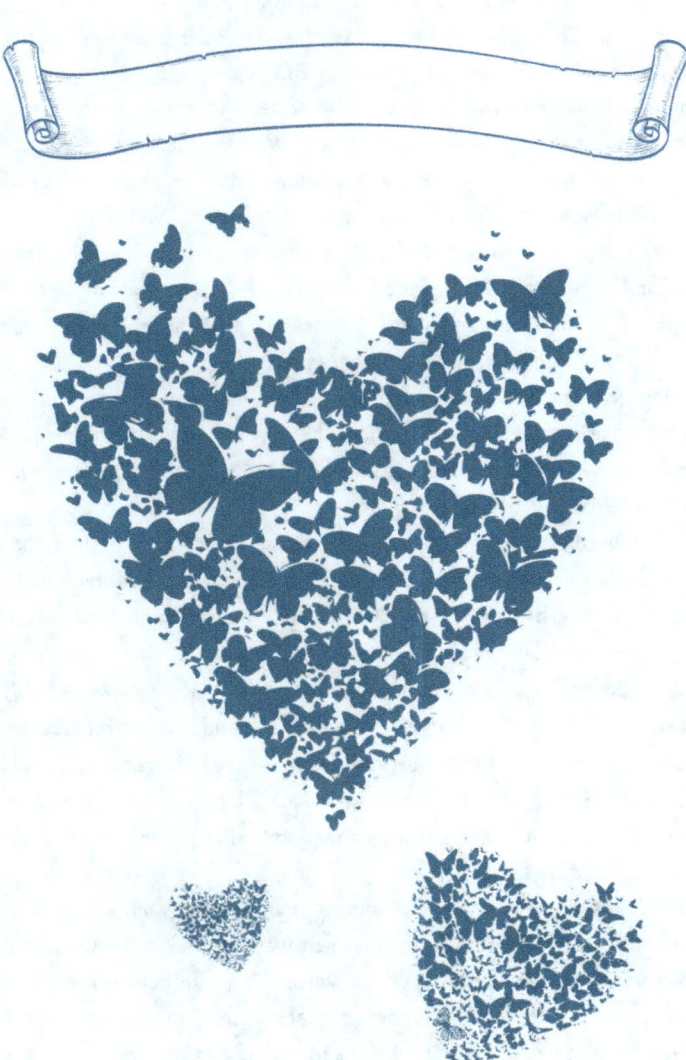

Swept Up

I visualize being lost at sea in the midst of a storm as I journey through grief. I have always loved the water. Even in my youth, I was dangerously fearless. It would be the fall of 1995 and my senior year of college studying abroad when my feet pressed into the warm sand of the Gold Coast. I gazed out at the Atlantic and the endless waters separating me from my family while I lived out my dream to live and study in Africa.

My time in Ghana, West Africa gave me far more than I anticipated. My first day held a lesson I wouldn't use for 30 years, but a lesson that would save my life. I couldn't wait to get in the waters of my ancestors, honor the lives lost in the Middle Passage, and forge new paths with my studies.

Stepping in was like entering a passageway to the mysteries of all that lay ahead. The waves crashed against my abdomen and I welcomed each one. I was fully in the moment and didn't notice the locals watching me with concern and confusion as I waded deeper. I felt a sudden drop in the temperature at my feet and when I took the next step, I sank under the water... the floor had vanished from beneath me.

Kicking until my head reached the surface, I had just enough time to take a breath before a wave crashed down on me and took my entire body. A soft whisper from within told me not to fight and to try to be one with the water. In reality, I didn't have a choice.

I was flipped, turned on my side, rolled one direction and then the other when suddenly it felt as if the Atlantic's hands grabbed my ankles and dragged me to the bottom of the ocean floor. As she pulled me out to sea, rocks and shells cut into my legs, bottom, and back.

It all happened in a split second, but for me the seconds were as vast as the ocean itself. When she finally released me and the waters calmed, my head surfaced and I gasped for air. All of my senses cleared and I could hear voices and shouting from the shore. The locals I passed on my way in were calling to me and I could see cupped hands gesturing for me to return. They were so small and so far away.

I felt sand bulging in the bottom of my swimsuit and my eyes burned from the salt, but I could still see the men waving me in. They had so much concern. I imagined the fins of a great white easing up behind me. Thoughts flooded my mind... then I remembered hearing that most accidents in the water happen when people panic. I decided to stay calm (and not look behind me for shark fins).

I focused on the shore, but from the corner of my eye I could see another huge wave approaching. With a peace I cannot explain, I pictured Mama in the water jumping waves. "Just, ride the wave, Marya." It was too deep and there was nothing I could use to kick off, so I did my best to thrust my body into the wave and move with it to the shore. I imagined myself as a dolphin who understood the waters' mood and ways.

Every wave took me a little closer ... but I kept time with her over and over again, slowly but surely inching closer to the shore. As I fought my way back, doubt crept in. I was so tired — I honestly didn't know if I would survive my fight with the Atlantic. She was an unpredictable force I could not contend with unless I listened to her and released — unless I submitted to her movements. I would not win a fight against her, but I could win a fight with her.

I crept toward the coast with each wave and then flattening my body on top of the water so not to be thrust back out or pulled under. Our dance went on this way for what felt like hours before I finally reached the shore.

So it has been with my grief journey — moments, days, months, and years I wasn't certain that I would survive. Grief swept me under the waters with just as much force as the Atlantic in my early twenties. My thirty minute battle at sea prepared me for my three years of grief... almost thirty years later.

The shock of my brother's death was as sudden as the wave and undertow. I was in bliss, living out a youthful spiritual sojourn... when out of nowhere, I was snatched. So was James. He was snatched — there one moment, gone the next. No explanation. Just gone.

~ Had I fought or panicked in the ocean, I wouldn't have survived. Her power was too strong.

~ Had I given up and completely succumbed to her strength, I wouldn't have survived. She would have taken me out to sea.

~ Had I been too strong, stubborn, or rigid, I wouldn't have survived. I was completely at her mercy.

The key was knowing when to release and when to fight against the water rushing at me, when to breathe and when to hold my breath. When to wipe my eyes and when to keep them shut and feel her movement and rhythm.

Surviving grief calls you to stand firm in truth and spirit... and to fight. I thank the wide open waters of the Atlantic Ocean for teaching me how.

Grief Comes
From Many Kinds of Loss

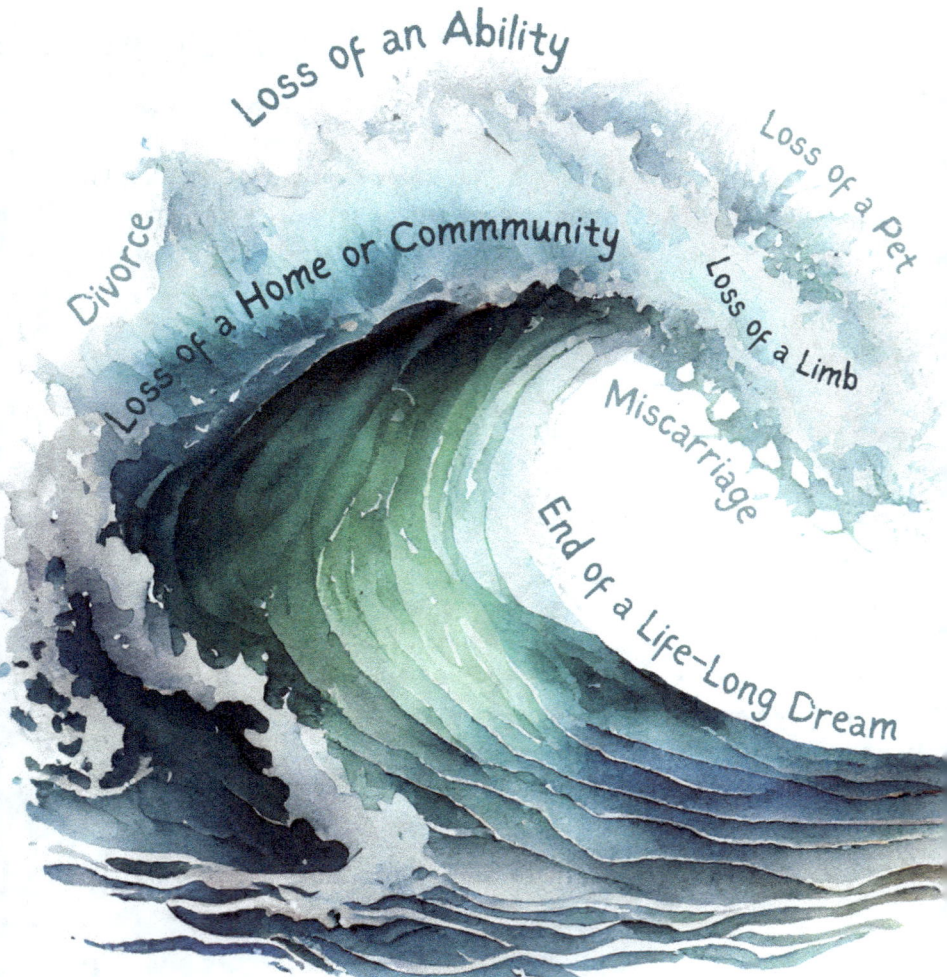

Death of a Loved One...

Loss of an Ability

Loss of a Pet

Divorce

Loss of a Home or Community

Loss of a Limb

Miscarriage

End of a Life-Long Dream

You Are Welcome Here

I have learned so much about grief — yet I know very little. This book is not advice and certainly not answers. I had several goals in mind when I began this project:

Provide Space: I'm a firm believer that less is very often more. The last thing many want are more words, more advice, and more "you shoulds." We all need to talk less and listen more. How often we deeply desire someone to ask us how we are and genuinely care enough to listen to our honest response. My hope is for "Into the Water" to offer you space to reflect, pray, rant, color, design, create, laugh, cry, and heal ~ space for what you need in your moment of need... space for your journey to be your own.

Share: For those interested in the journey, experiences, and thoughts of others, I invite you to take part in the experiences of others who selflessly share part of their walk. Each one of us will experience grief differently ~ as we should, but we can also learn from each other if we are open to doing so.

Encourage: I'm a fixer to a fault as my family knows all too well. It takes prayer and great restraint to stop and listen rather than jump in and do. Often times, what others need from us is to merely listen, be present, and allow them to share their struggles without a quick-fix being thrown at them. My hope is to encourage you as you process and gently remind you that you are deeply loved & most assuredly not alone.

A year into my grief journey, I was drowning. I could not get a hold of my emotions and the daily mood swings. I felt like I was failing myself, failing my family, and frankly, on the edge of crash and burn. A sweet friend listened patiently and said it sounded like I was experiencing all the stages of grief daily. Stages of Grief? I read everything I could to better understand myself, but Elisabeth Kübler-Ross' book, "On Death and Dying" was the most helpful. "Into the Water" is broken into 7 sections to reflect 7 stages of grief.

May you find Space here, gain something from those who opted to Share, and may you be Encouraged in knowing that our Lord's love is infinite and sufficient.

Love & Prayers Always,
Marya

shock

Not everyone experiences shock. The circumstances of loss and the kind of loss are both a factor. For many, shock is difficult to avoid even if we had prior knowledge and time to prepare.

Shock looks different for everyone, but very often, we continue naturally with routines and may appear emotionless. Our feeling can be too intense for our minds and hearts to fully process.

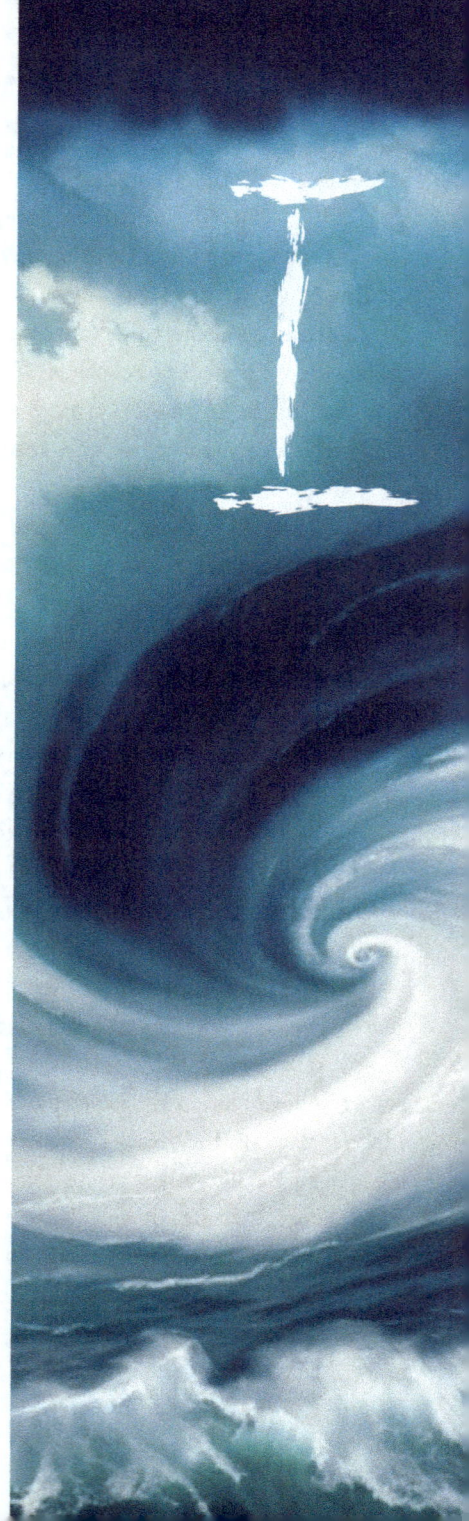

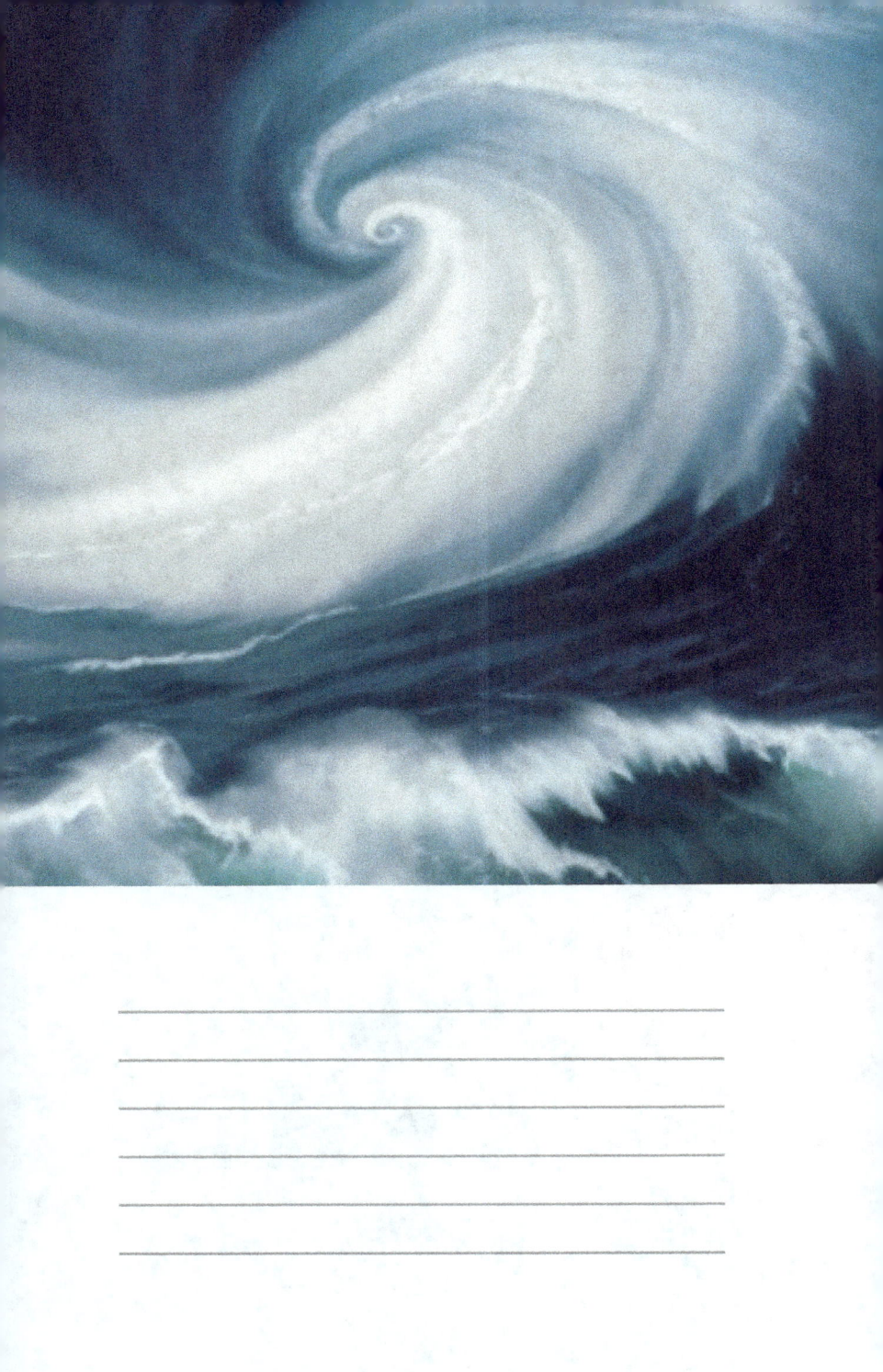

_____

_____

_____

_____

_____

_____

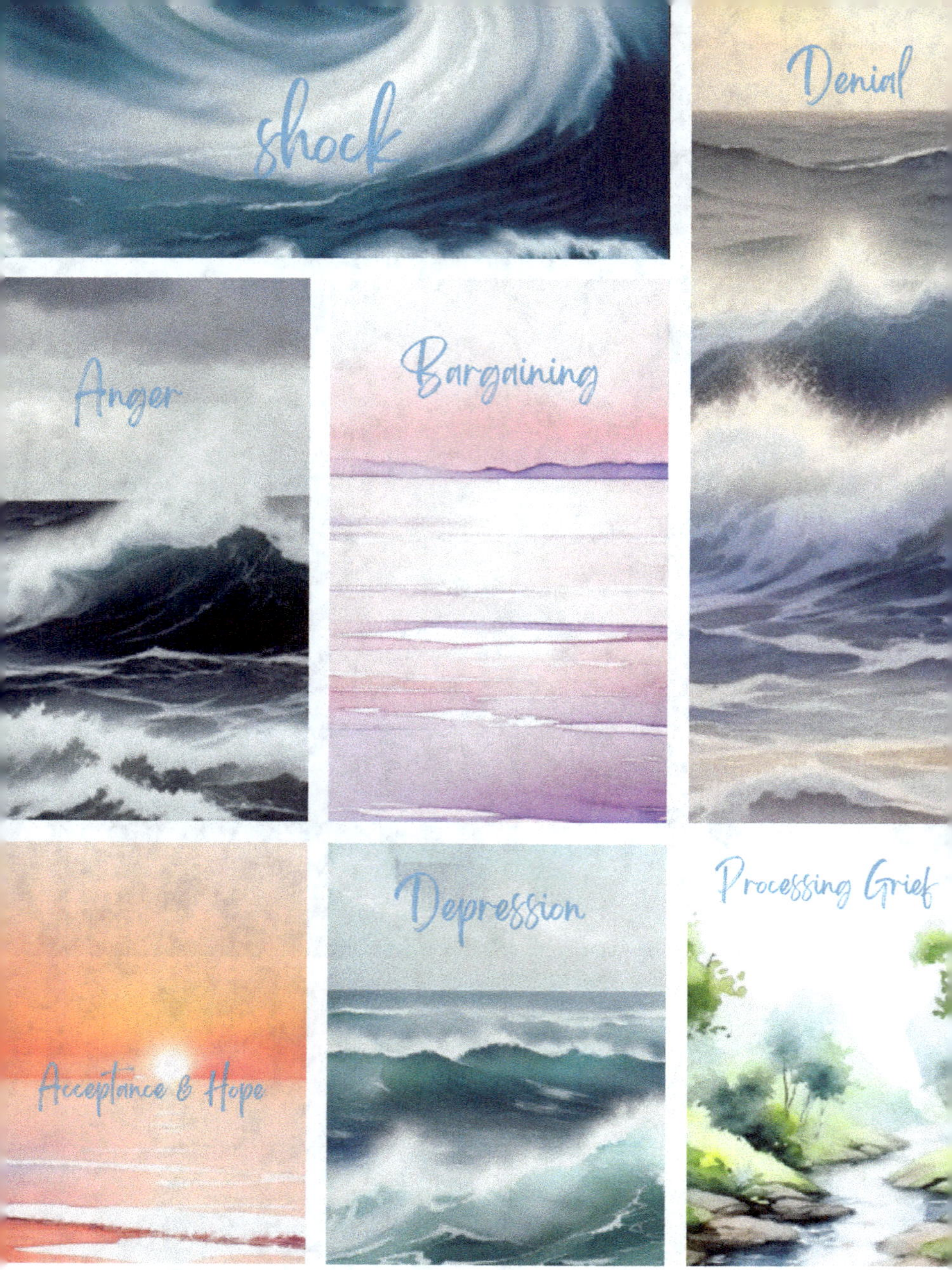

shock

Denial

Anger

Bargaining

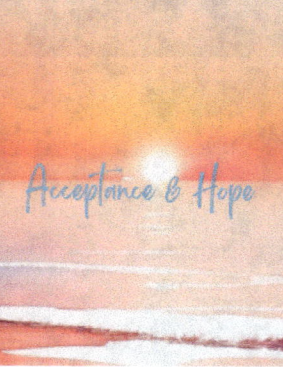

Acceptance & Hope

Depression

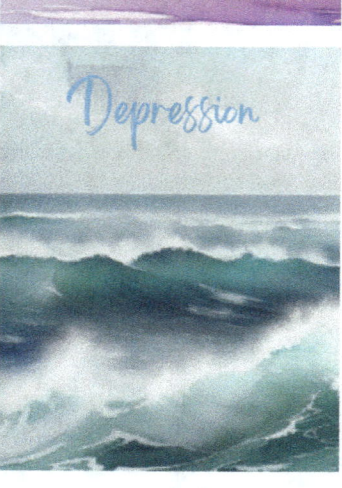

Processing Grief

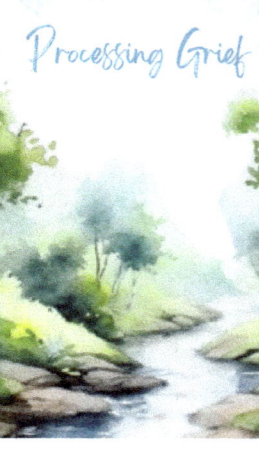

Where Are You Today?

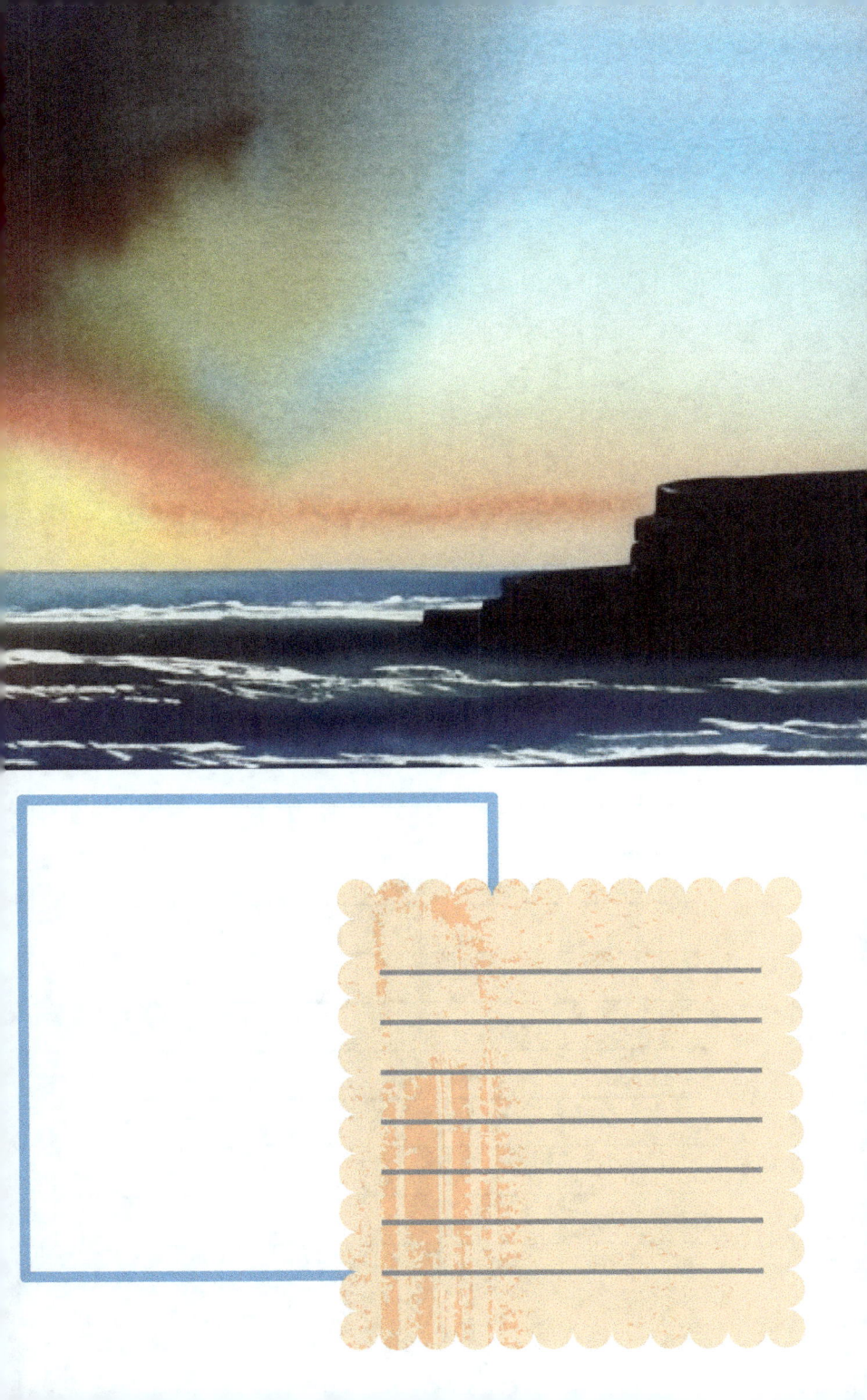

Check-In

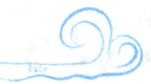

It is important to Be where you Are. Reflect on your dominant emotions and what's captivating your mind? What is your greatest need right now?

_____

_____

_____

_____

_____

_____

_____

_____

_____

_____

_____

Possible Prompts

How have you been eating & sleeping?

What brings you the most comfort right now?

Do you feel like you need to hide your grief or
can your grieve genuinely?

Who could you have lunch or coffee with that
would bring you comfort?

Have you given yourself permission to walk
through the grieving process?

Describe your inner circle — who can you lean
on to support you and in what specific ways?

What role has shock played?

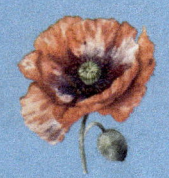

Thoughts on Grief

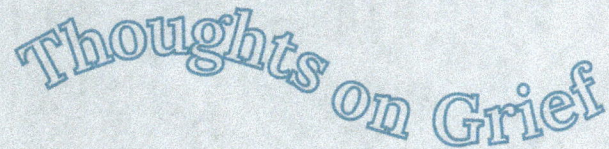

The following quotes are never far from my mind. They remind me my grief is not an isolated story of pain. I'm never alone, and that I've overcome 100% of the trials, tragedies, traumas, and difficult times in my life so far. Every day I choose to KEEP GOING.

~ Marissa

Never, never, never give up.
~ Winston Churchill

Fall down seven times, stand up eight.
~ Japanese Proverb

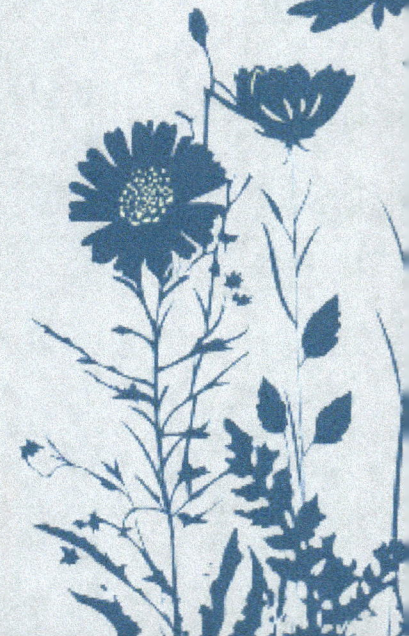

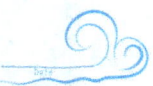

Date

Blessed are those who mourn.
for they will be comforted.

Matthew 5:4

Date

_____

_____

_____

_____

_____

_____

_____

_____

_____

_____

_____

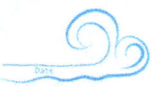

So do not fear, for I am with you; do not
be dismayed, for I am your God. I will
strengthen you and help you; I will uphold
you with my righteous right hand.

Isaiah 41:10

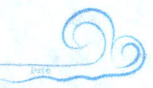

Self-Care Check

Exercise & Activities

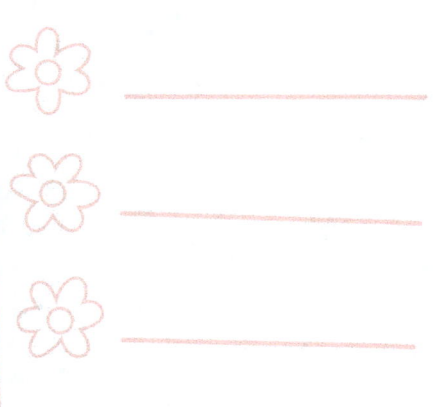

How much
water did you
drink today?

What was the best
part of your day?

Who are you grateful
for? Who or what made
a difference in your day?

Letter to My Future Self

Instructions are on the following page.

Dear   ,

_____

_____

_____

_____

_____

_____

_____

_____

_____

Love,

Date:

Dear Self...

The previous page is here for you to consider where you would like to be when you conclude this book (keeping in mind that you should work at your own pace). Expressing where you currently Are and where you want to Be in the future is casting a vision. In doing this, we are fueling our movement with hope.

There are no right or wrong answers... no one knows You better than You. See yourself in the future and describe all you see - your growth and healing. Imagine your victories and don't be afraid to think Big. Be Bold. Be Adventurous.

Be Hope.

I can do all this through him who gives me strength.

Philippians 4:13

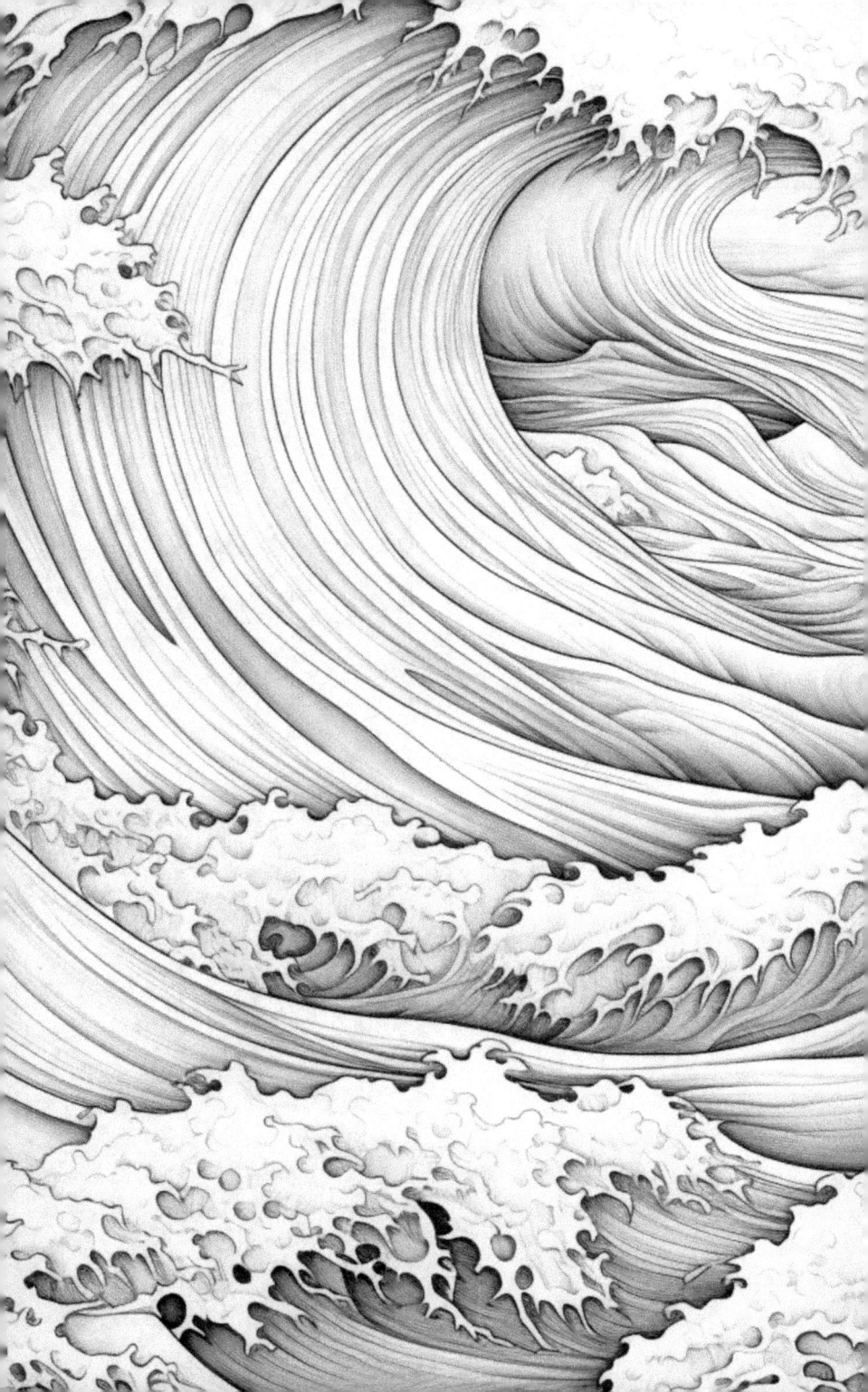

Denial

Denial crept in because it felt familiar — like shock's distant cousin.

Prior to experiencing denial, it carried a negative connotation in my mind, but I am now grateful for the respite denial offered. Don't get me wrong, denial is not a healthy place to live, but it gave me time.

For me, Denial was an intuitive survival technique that kicked in and remained until I was ready to face the truth that lay ahead.

We can all agree that denial is not the end goal, but do not allow guilt to set in if you walk through this stage.

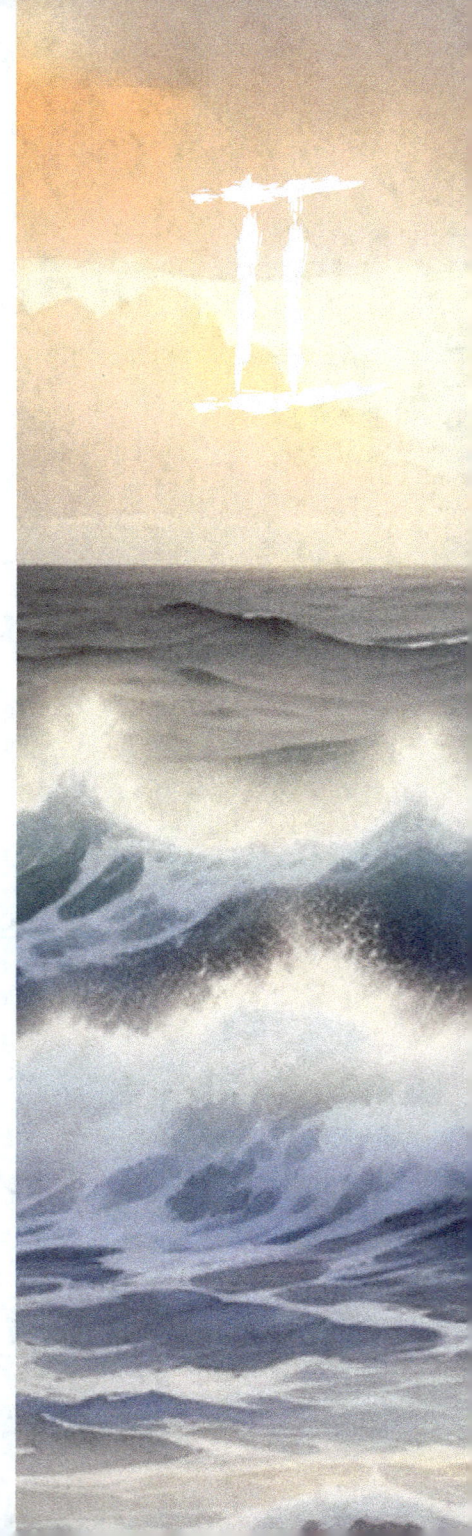

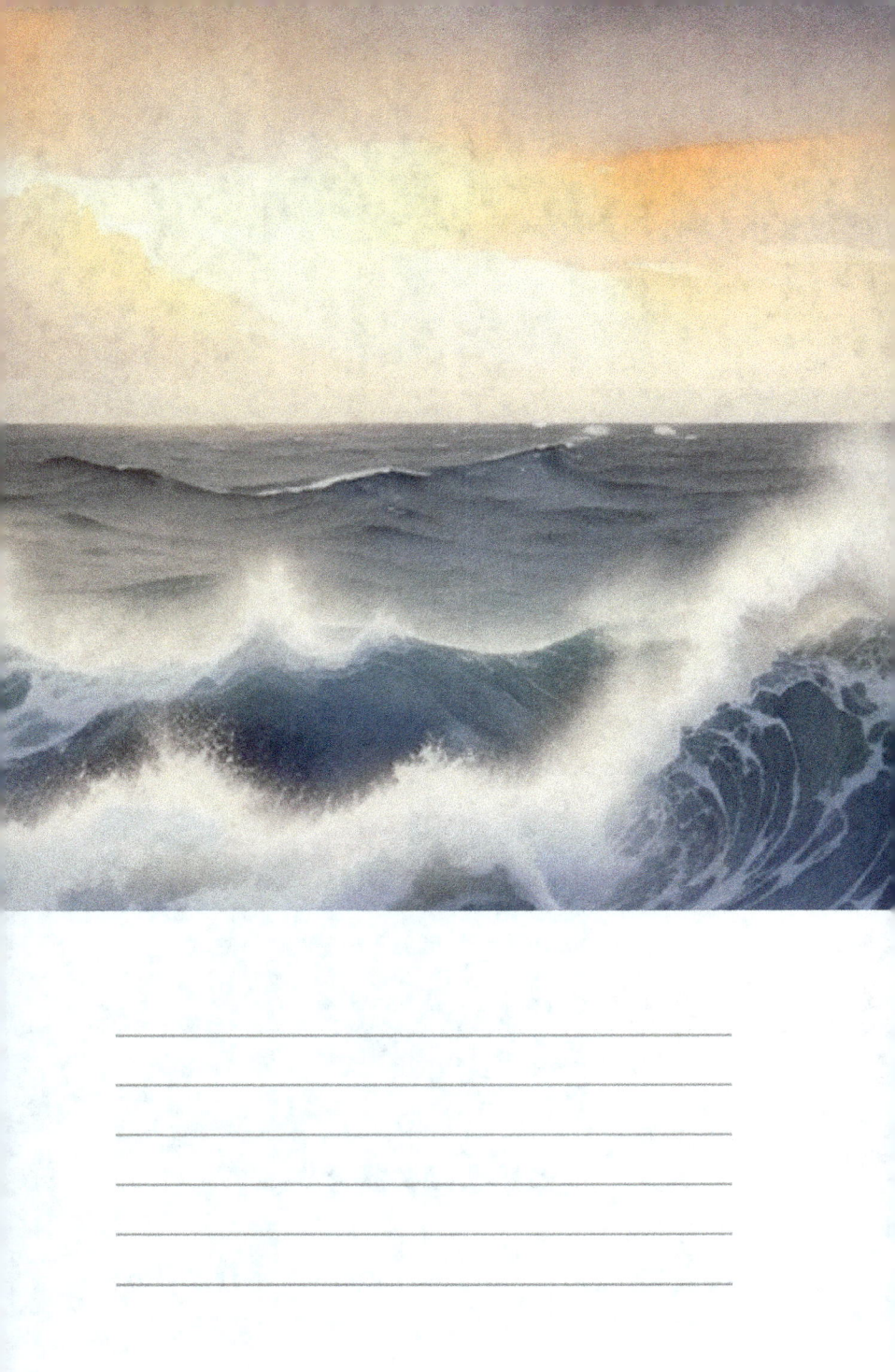

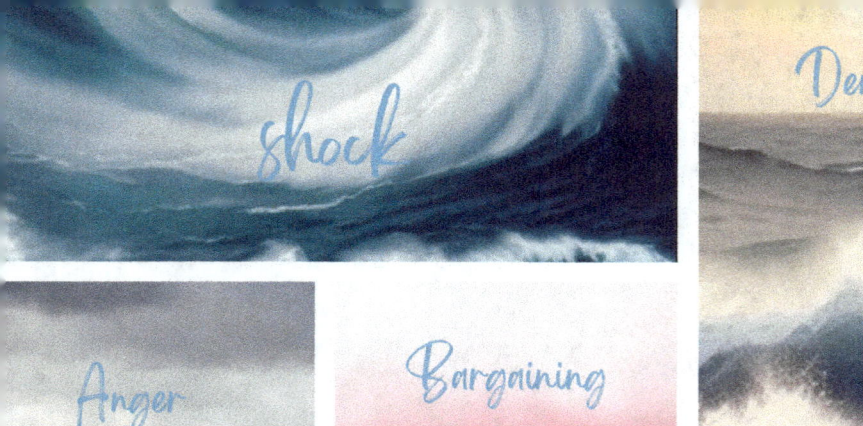

shock

Denial

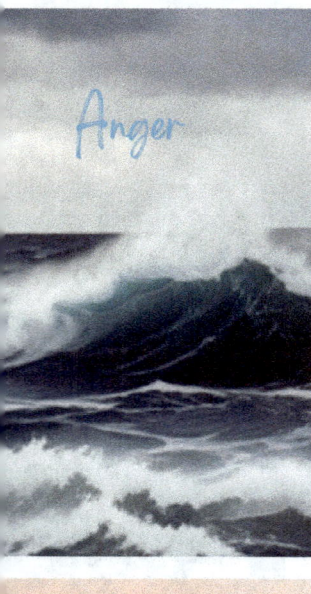

Anger

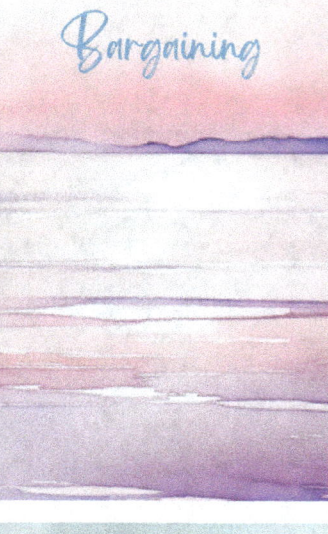

Bargaining

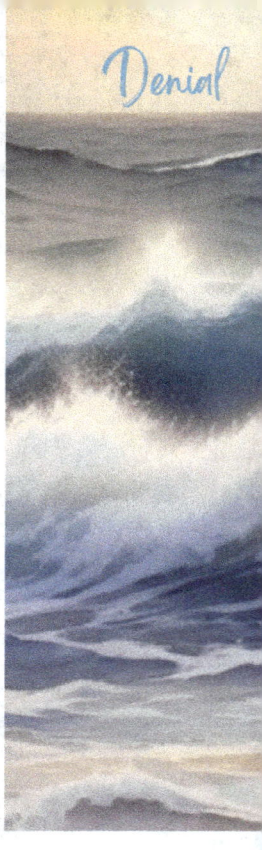

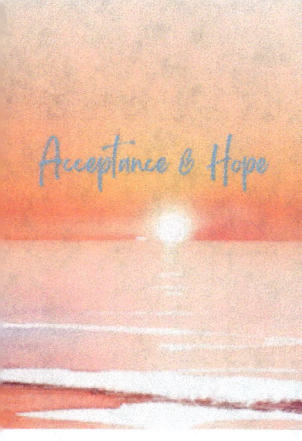

Acceptance & Hope

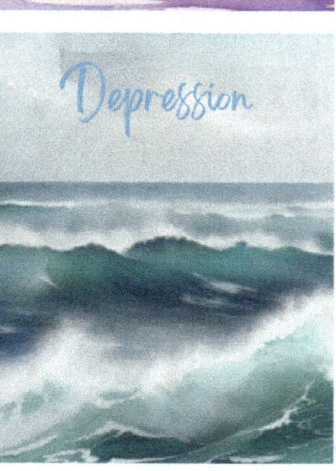

Depression

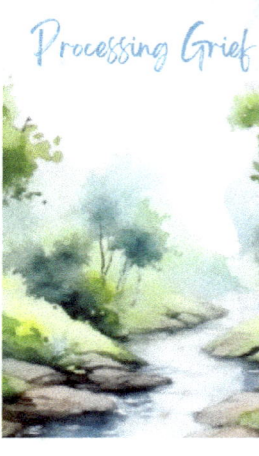

Processing Grief

Where Are You Today?

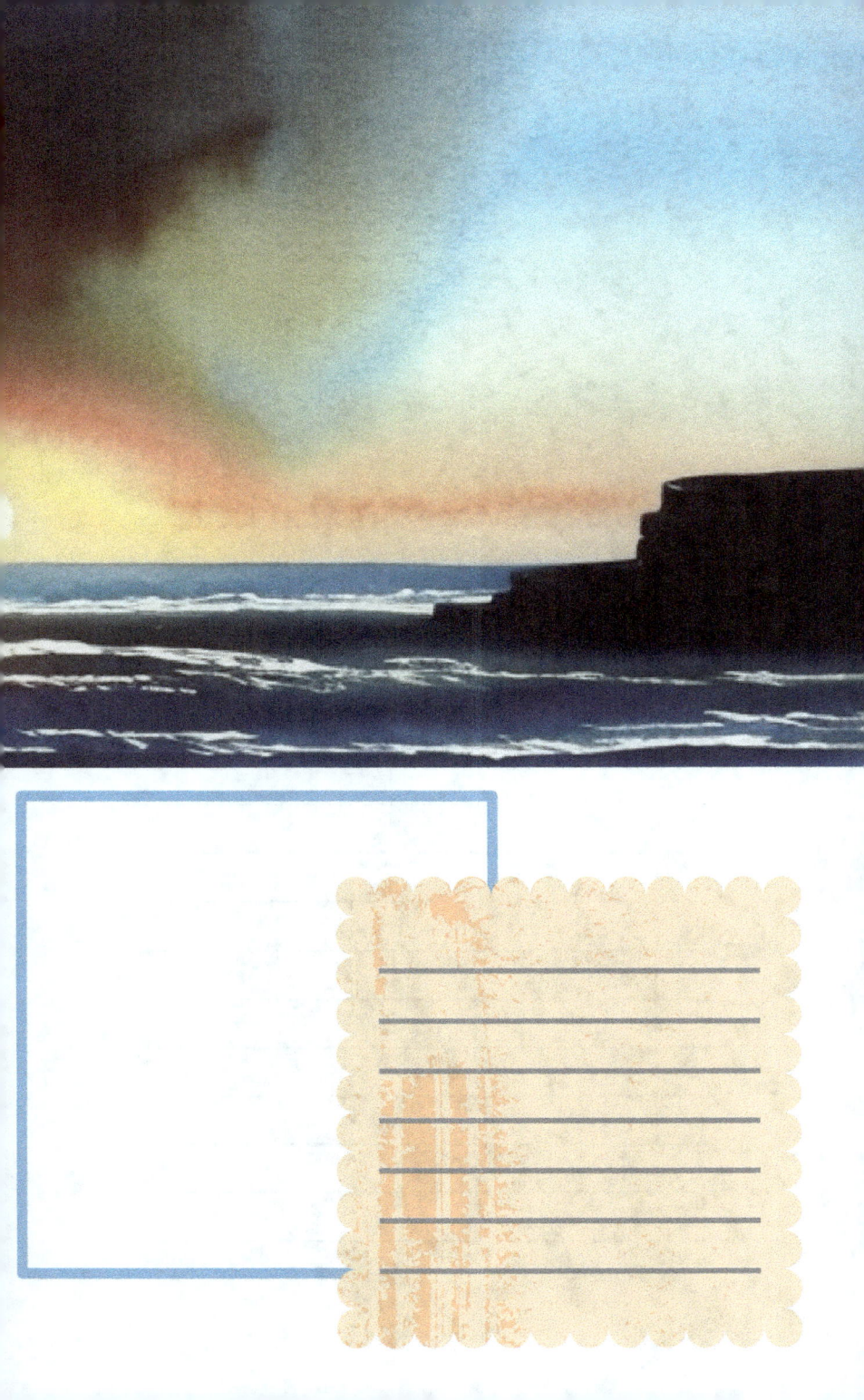

Check-In

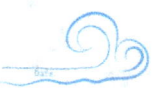

Remember to Be where you Are.
Reflect on your dominant
emotions and what's captivating
your mind? What is your
greatest need right now?

_____
_____
_____
_____
_____
_____
_____
_____
_____
_____

Possible Prompts

Have you shared your story and feelings —
have you released?

In what ways can you be more patient with
yourself?

Have you given yourself permission to heal in
your own way and at your own pace?

What are ways you can politely quiet those
who attempt to rush or define your journey?

What have you not spoken or put to words
that you desperately need to say or write?

What are your greatest needs at this
moment?

What challenges and good could come to pass if
you acknowledge this loss?

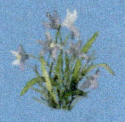

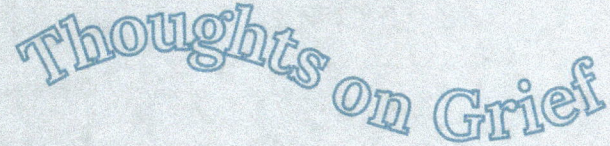

Thoughts on Grief

Michelle Nelson Kuzma shared this beautiful passage...

As for grief, you'll find it comes in waves. When the ship is first wrecked, you're drowning, with wreckage all around you. Everything floating around you reminds you of the beauty and the magnificence of the ship that was, and is no more. And all you can do is float. You find some piece of the wreckage and you hang on for a while. Maybe it's some physical thing. Maybe it's a happy memory or a photograph. Maybe it's a person who is also floating. For a while, all you can do is float. Stay alive. In the beginning, the waves are 100 feet tall and crash over you without mercy. They come 10 seconds apart and don't even give you time to catch your breath. All you can do is hang on and float. After a while, maybe weeks, maybe months, you'll find the waves are still 100 feet tall, but they come further apart. When they come, they still crash all over you and wipe you out. But in between, you can breathe, you can function.

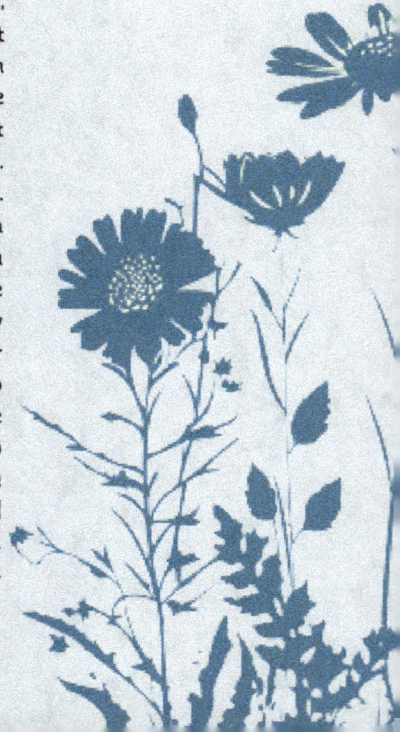

You never know what's going to trigger the grief. It might be a song, a picture, a street intersection, the smell of a cup of coffee. It can be just about anything...and the wave comes crashing. But in between waves, there is life. Somewhere down the line, and it's different for everybody, you find that the waves are only 80 feet tall. Or 50 feet tall. And while they still come, they come further apart. You can see them coming. An anniversary, a birthday, or Christmas, or landing at O'Hare. You can see it coming, for the most part, and prepare yourself. And when it washes over you, you know that somehow you will, again, come out the other side. Soaking wet, sputtering, still hanging on to some tiny piece of the wreckage, but you'll come out. Take it from an old guy. The waves never stop coming, and somehow you don't really want them to. But you learn that you'll survive them. And other waves will come. And you'll survive them too. If you're lucky, you'll have lots of scars from lots of loves. And lots of shipwrecks.

~ excerpt from Reddit, GSnow

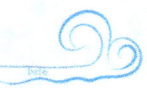

He will wipe every tear from their eyes.
There will be no more death or mourning
or crying or pain, for the old order
of things has passed away.

Revelation 21:4

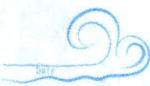

Only people who are capable of loving
strongly can also suffer great sorrow,
but this same necessity of loving
serves to counteract their grief and heal them.

~ Leo Tolstoy

_____
_____
_____
_____
_____
_____
_____
_____
_____
_____

Find your special place to spend time alone with our Lord regularly.

Car, prayer closet, on a walk, a park, or in your mind's eye
– the place does not matter.
Be with Him.

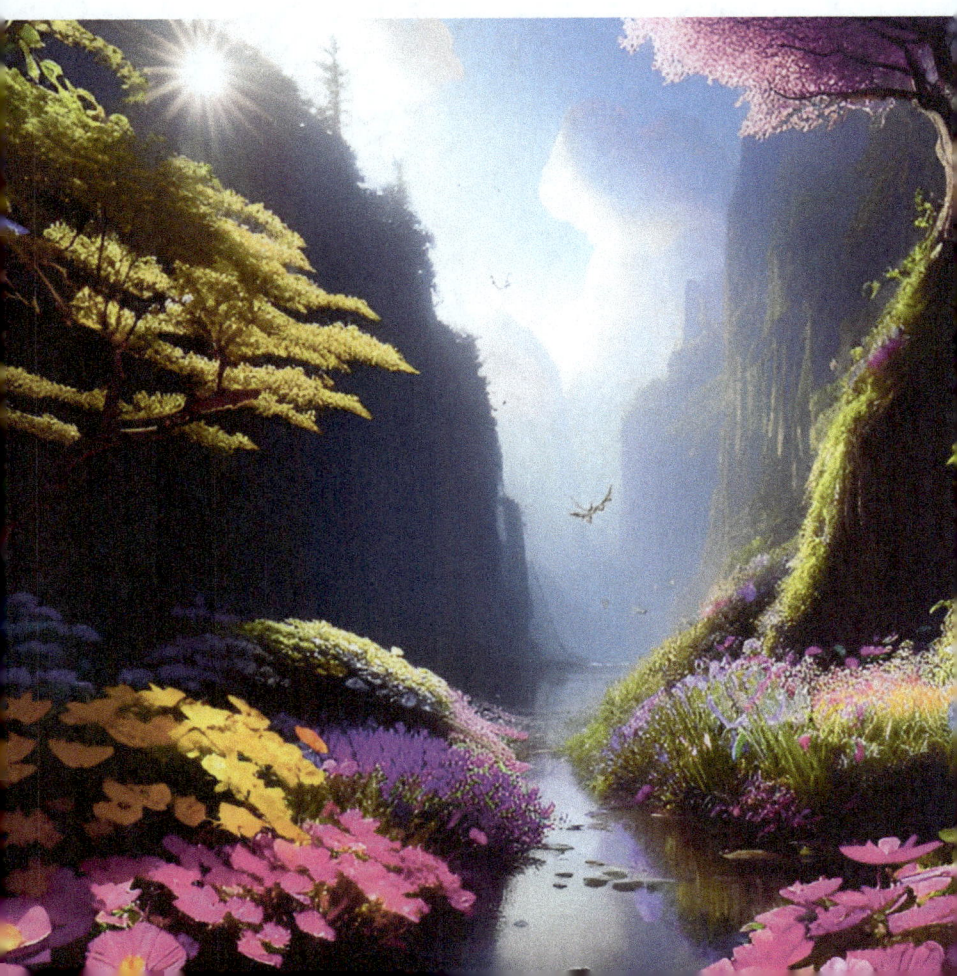

Self-Care Check

Exercise & Activities

How much water did you drink today?

What was the best part of your day?

Who are you grateful for? Who or what made a difference in your day?

Overcoming Grief by Navigating the Grief Continuum

by David A. Sherron

"Consider it pure joy, my brothers and sisters, whenever you face trials of many kinds, because you know that the testing of your faith produces perseverance. Let perseverance finish its work so that you may be mature and complete, not lacking anything."
James 1: 2-4

The biggest mistake most of us make is that we rush through our grief. Our grief has a purpose and benefit, neither of which can be revealed and executed unless our grief is completely cycled through.

Let's explore the purpose and benefit of our grief by examining each component of the grief cycle through the grief continuum (which moves you from bondage to grief, to freedom from grief): Bondage to Grief, Freedom from Grief, Acknowledge Grief, Accept Grief, Embrace Grief, Explore Grief, and Release Grief.

Bondage to Grief ⟹ Freedom from Grief ⟹ Acknowledge Grief ⟹ Accept Grief ⟹ Embrace Grief ⟹ Explore Grief ⟹ Release Grief.

<u>Acknowledging Grief</u>: Call out your grief, don't pretend it away. Grief doesn't have to be justified, rationalized, vetted, confirmed, or verified. When grief enters the room don't ignore it like it's not there. Welcome grief, invite it to have a seat and relax. After all, grief might be staying for a while.

"I have told you these things, so that in me you may have peace. In this world you will have trouble. But take heart! I have overcome the world."
John 16:33

<u>Accept Grief</u>: Grief is nothing to be ashamed of, grief is not a sign of weakness, grief is not a social stigma. Tell your grief that you have no fear of it, that you are not intimidated by it, and that you are quite familiar with it.

"Dear friends, do not be surprised at the fiery ordeal that has come on you to test you, as though something strange were happening to you."
1 Peter 4:12

<u>Embrace Grief:</u> Understand that grief – like joy, pain, triumph, and defeat – is a natural part of life. Grief is not to be shunned or denied, that only prolongs the grieving process. Grief is to be embraced, just as we embrace the continuous cycle of seasons. Think of grief the same way you think of the coldest days of winter – it comes periodically, it lasts for a time, and then it eventually gives way to the brighter days of spring.

"In all this you greatly rejoice, though now for a little while you may have had to suffer grief in all kinds of trials. These have come so that the proven genuineness of your faith–of greater worth than gold, which perishes even though refined by fire–may result in praise, glory and honor when Jesus Christ is revealed." 1 Peter 1: 6–7

<u>Explore Grief:</u> Rather than rush through your grief, explore it. Be curious about your grief. Treat your grief like your child's best friend whom you happen to dislike – it may not be desirable, but since it's going to be in your life you might as well get to know it.

"Trust in the Lord with all your heart and lean not on your own understanding; in all your ways submit to him, and he will make your paths straight." Proverbs 3: 5–6

<u>Release Grief:</u> Like an old pair of shoes that no longer fit, at some point it's time to tell your grief goodbye. Only you will know exactly when. However, when your grief no longer has utility, meaning, and purpose – when you start wearing your grief as a badge of honor rather than bridge to higher ground. When you find your grief sitting in your lounge chair with its feet propped up on your coffee table, while watching your TV and eating up your munchies, then your grief has probably gotten too comfortable in your life – time to show your grief the door!

"The righteous cry out, and the Lord hears them; he delivers them from all their troubles. The Lord is close to the brokenhearted and saves those who are crushed in spirit." Psalms 34: 17–18

One last thing. As previous revealed, your grief has purpose and benefit... but for whom? The fruit of your grief may not be intended for your own personal gain. Who is watching how you navigate through your grief? Who is learning from your example, and now being prepared for their next struggle with grief as a result? Who is now successfully managing their current bout with grief because of the comfort you are providing them through your own credible testimony?

"Praise be to the God and Father of our Lord Jesus Christ, the Father of compassion and the God of all comfort, who comforts us in all our troubles, so that we can comfort those in any trouble with the comfort we ourselves receive from God." 2 Corinthians 1:3–4

Anger

Most of my life, my passion has been mistaken for anger. In truth, it takes a lot to make me angry. When I'm angry, I'm quiet. I'm taking the necessary steps to find myself so I won't do or say something I will regret. But anger is an emotion just like the others and should not be silenced, rushed, or benched. A time-out is not an effective approach if it causes you to stuff, mask, or hide your feelings.

I get it, anger can make others uncomfortable, just like grief. This is often because it is difficult to know what to say or not say, or how to respond. Even so, our anger is real and needs to be what it is while we work through it.

Be angry.

Don't stay angry.

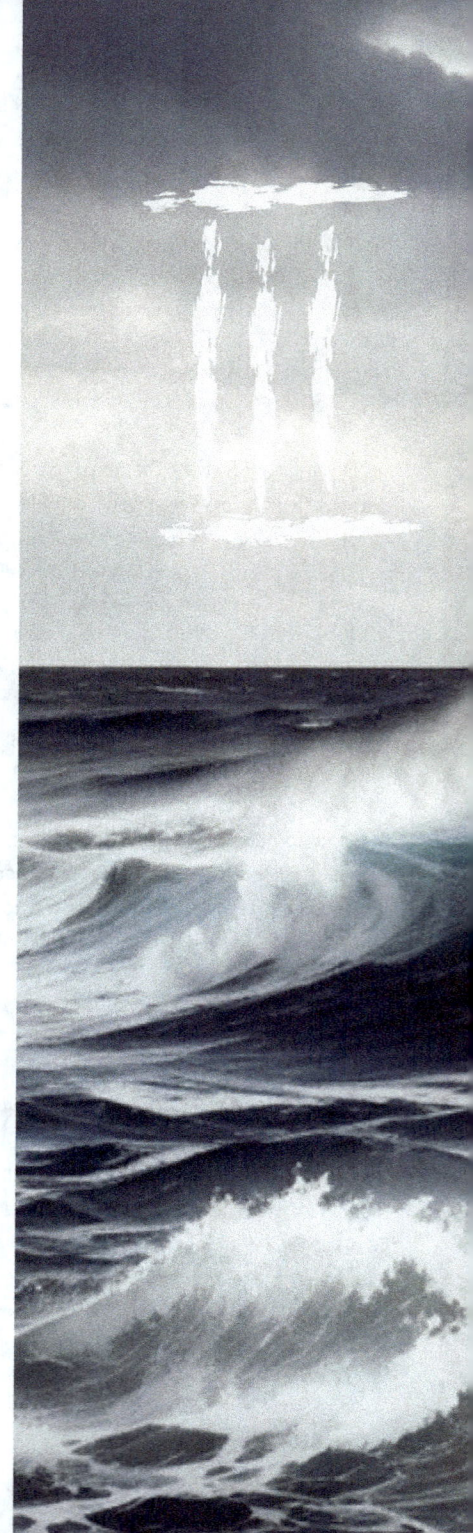

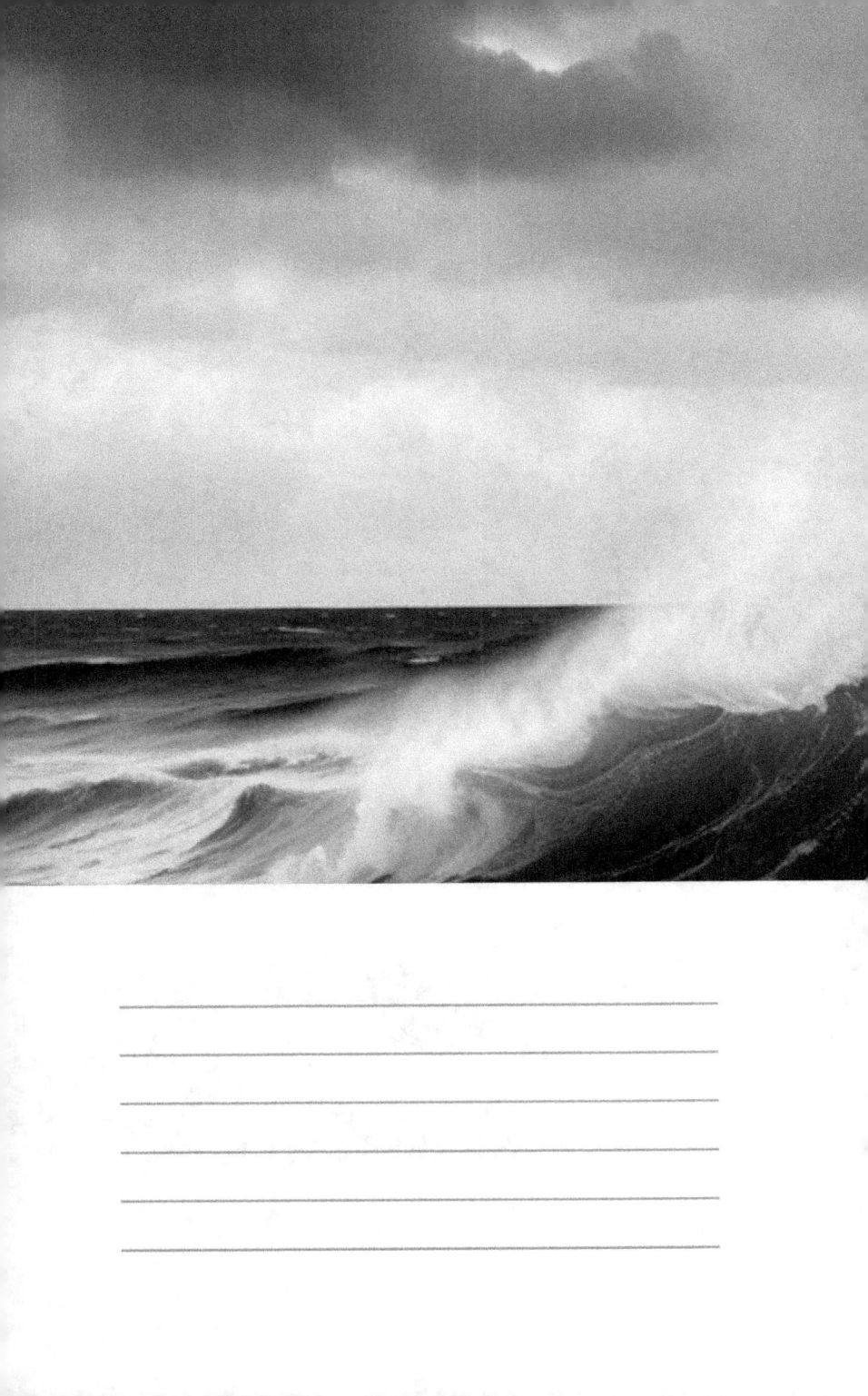

_____

_____

_____

_____

_____

_____

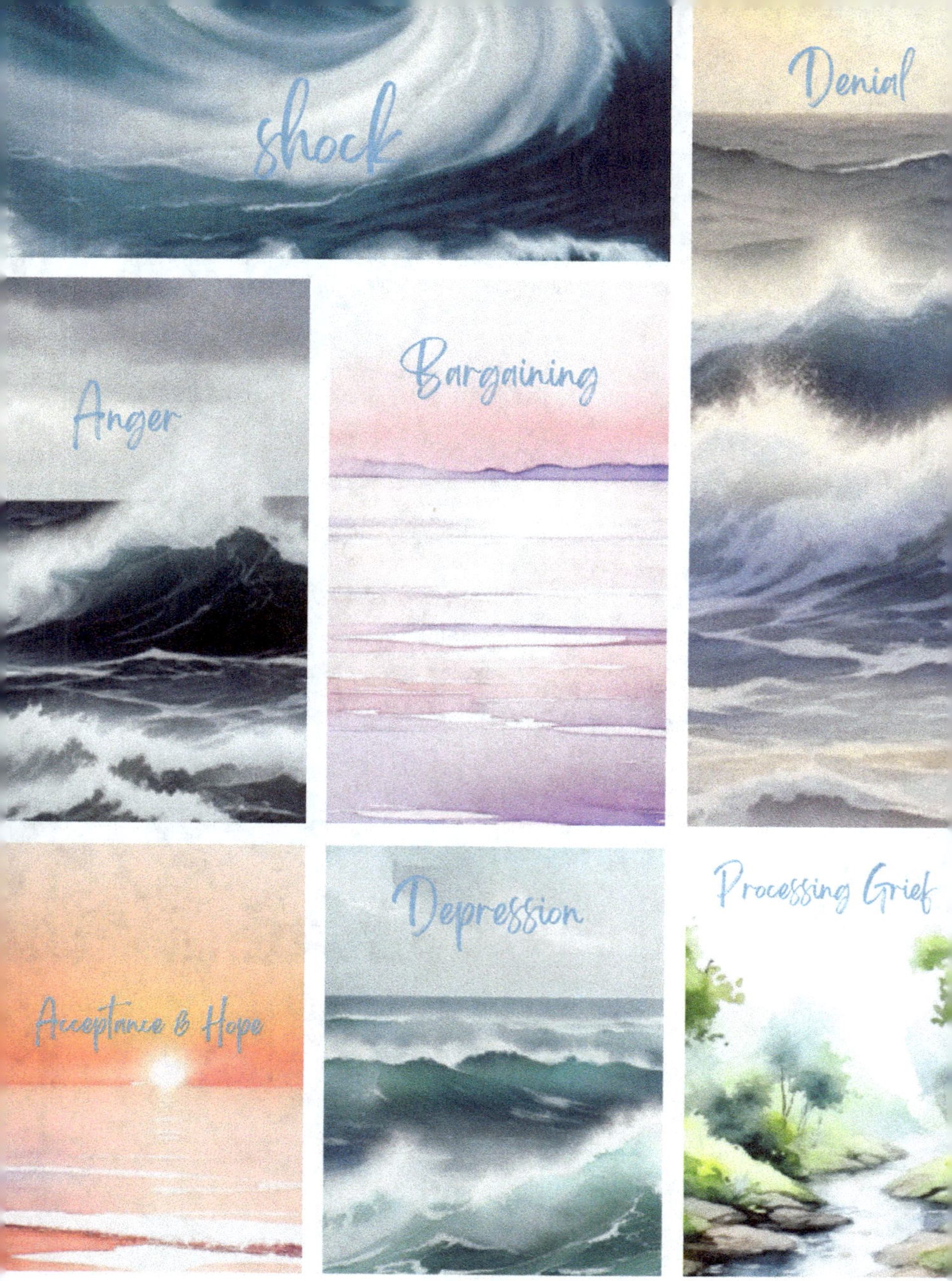

shock

Denial

Anger

Bargaining

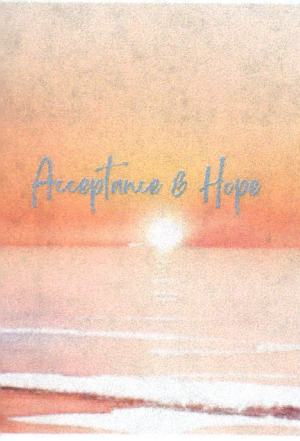

Acceptance & Hope

Depression

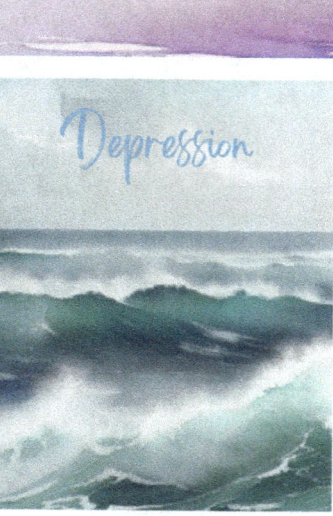

Processing Grief

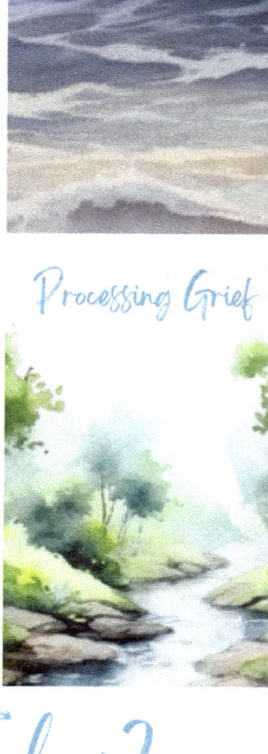

Where Are You Today?

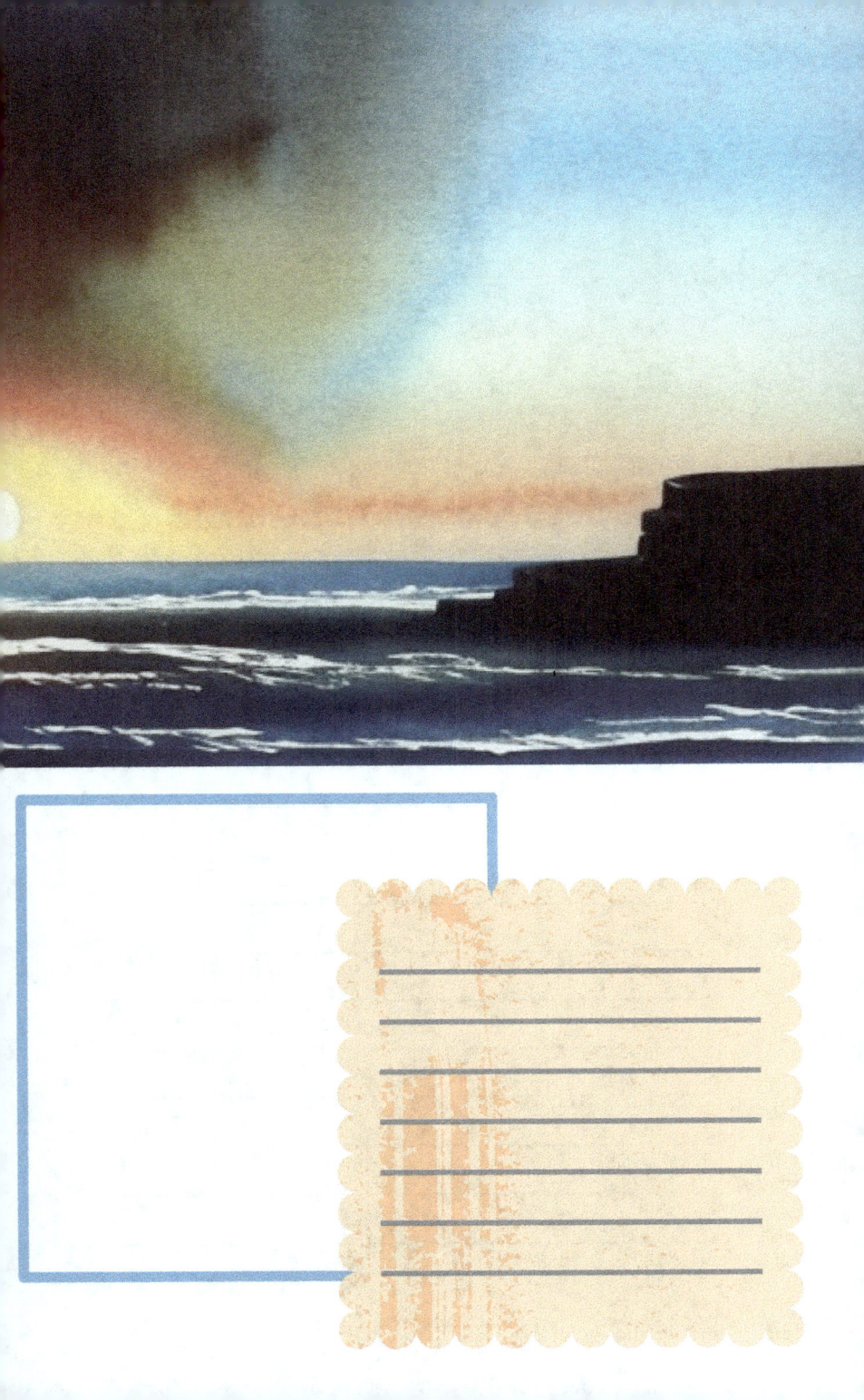

Check-In

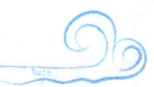

Remember to Be where you Are.
Reflect on your dominant
emotions and what's captivating
your mind? What is your
greatest need right now?

_____

_____

_____

_____

_____

_____

_____

_____

_____

_____

Possible Prompts

What situations, places, or words currently invoke anger?

Pass your anger the mic —write down all it has to say?

If you could replace anger with a different emotion, what would it be?

Anger isn't bad, it's one of our many emotions and completely natural. However, living in anger can cause stress and eventually affect your overall health. Think about calming techniques and what helps you move through and beyond anger.

Write a rant or list all of the things that make you angry — then burn it.

Are there places, people, or entities you should avoid with regard to anger?

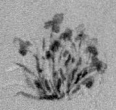

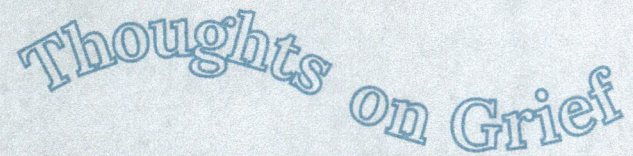

There are many types of loss. Some are sudden, where you are caught off guard and didn't have a chance to get closure. Those wounds are deep.

There are other types of loss that are long goodbyes. Those wounds are deep too.

Your life experiences will shape the way you deal with grief. I've never lived your life and you haven't lived mine. That's why everyone deals with grief differently, in their own way.

Grief is a journey all humans take. We are all born into this world knowing someday we will exit it forever. Remember we are all humans. We grieve our losses in our own way, in our own time.

Avoid comparing your grief journey with another person's grief journey. Comparisons are not beneficial because we all handle grief differently. Comparisons will keep you stuck in the stage you are at. You'll never get to peace and acceptance by comparing your unique experience with someone else's unique experience.

It is okay to feel your feelings! It is okay to express your emotions! Just make sure you do so in a positive and healthy way that does not impede someone else's progress on their journey. It's okay if you need help to learn heathy behaviors. Ask for it.

Be open to the lessons you'll learn on your grief journey. You will learn so much about yourself. You'll also learn so much about others on your journey.

Although the journey is long, painful and difficult, it will get better. Your journey is unique to you, yet simultaneously a shared experience all humans will have. That's the interesting dichotomy of grief. You may be on your journey alone, but it's a journey we all take. It is the most human of all human experiences.

Do not make any major life decisions for one year after your loss. That means you should not marry someone, get a divorce, make financial decisions, change jobs, or adopt a pet until you have given yourself at least that amount of time to figure things out and adjust to your new normal. You owe it to yourself to take your time when navigating this journey. And most of all, you are worth it!

If you don't deal with your grief, your grief will deal with you. It will come out in ways you never imagined.

Be kind to yourself. You're worth that too!

~ Angela Miller

Brothers, we do not want you to be
ignorant about those who fall asleep,
or to grieve like the rest of men, who
have no hope.

1 Thessalonians 4:13

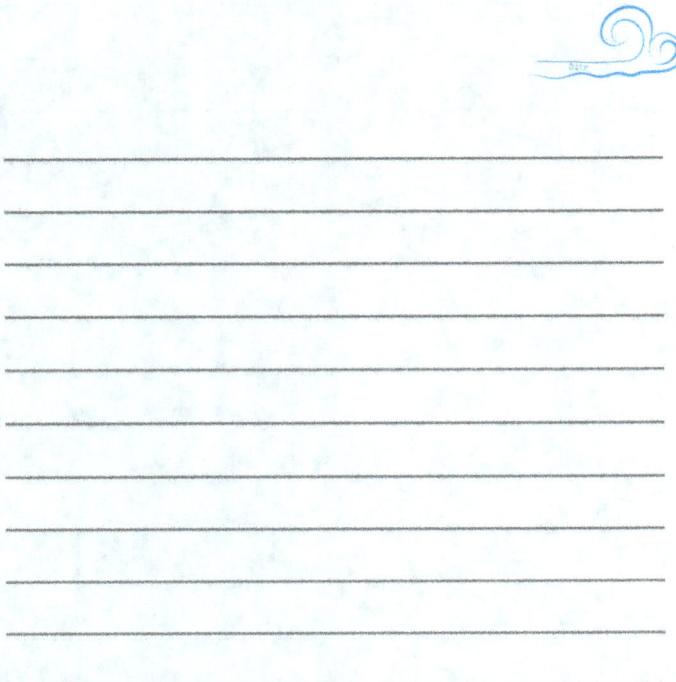

_____
_____
_____
_____
_____
_____
_____
_____
_____
_____
_____

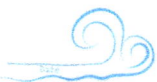

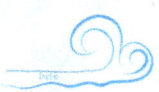

Jesus said to her, "I am the resurrection and the life. He who believes in me will live, even though he dies; and whoever lives and believes in me will never die. Do you believe this?

John 11:25-26

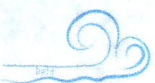

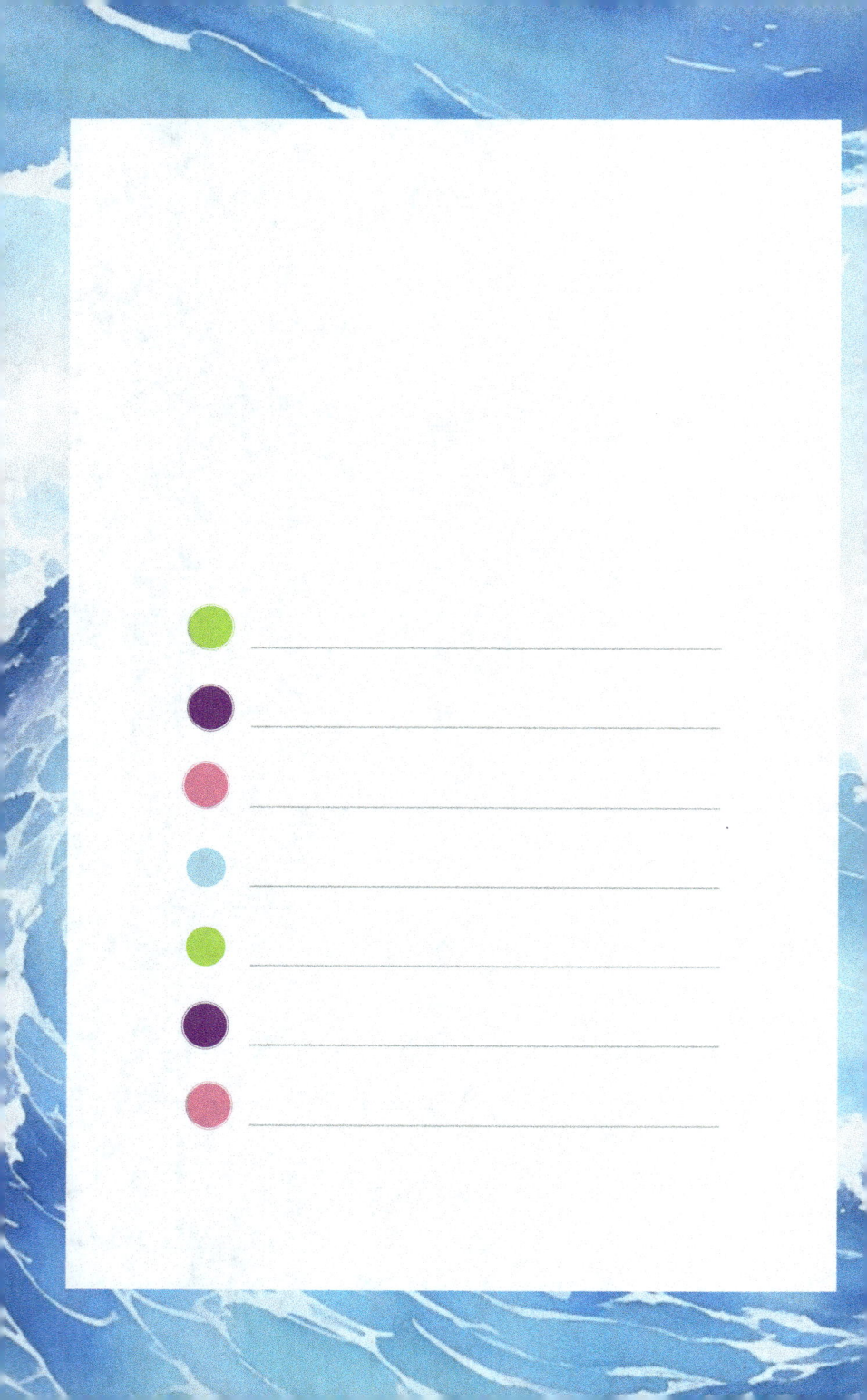

Self-Care Check

Exercise & Activities

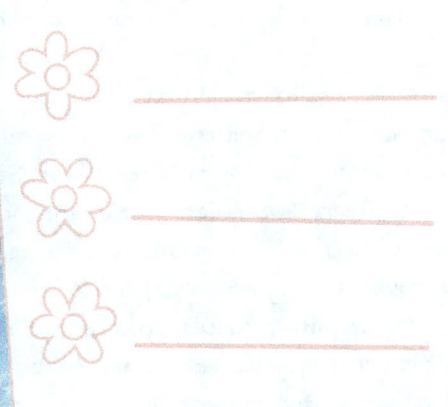

How much
water did you
drink today?

What was the best
part of your day?

Who are you grateful
for? Who or what made
a difference in your day?

What Grief and Loss Will Never Tell You
by Malika King

I'm no stranger to Grief and Loss. We first met when I was a young child. We're not friends, but I know them well. They have been more like unpredictable teachers without a syllabus or guidelines. They show up with one rule, you can't leave until you are ready. One of the things that makes Grief and Loss feel so heartless is how they will blindside you. They just show up when they want to, as if boundaries and the rest of your life doesn't exist. I must admit I'm not fond of these teachers, but I do respect them. I'm grateful for the lessons learned. I'm stronger, resilient, and wiser. I am also more broken, humble, and fragile. I'm complex, much like my teachers.

After repeated attempts, Grief and Loss has taught me that I have to run to God with all my pain. Run and sit. Run and cry. Run and scream. Run and question. Run and process. Rinse and repeat. When I hear God whisper, I must cherish it and obey. There is strength in His presence, enough life to get me to the next whisper. When I master this lesson, I fulfill James 1:2-4, "My brethren, count it all joy when you fall into various trials, knowing that the testing of your faith produces patience. But let patience have its perfect work, that you may be perfect and complete, lacking nothing." This means you too are invited to run to God in grief and trials, and He will perfect and mature you through it.

David is our example on what this process looks like in scripture. In I Samuel 30, David and his soldiers came back to the campgrounds, only to discover that their wives and children were kidnapped, their belongings were stolen, and their campgrounds were burned up. In their anger and grief, David's men blamed him as their leader. Not only was David having to process his own personal grief. He also had to carry the burden of others. David and his men were in so much emotional pain that it says that they "wept aloud until they had no strength left to weep" (I Samuel 30:4). David responded to grief by running to God with His pain, gaining strength at the feet of His Father, and asking Him for instructions that he obeyed.

David gives you the cliff notes that Grief and Loss will never dare tell you. It gives you an outline, but you still have to write your own story with the Lord.

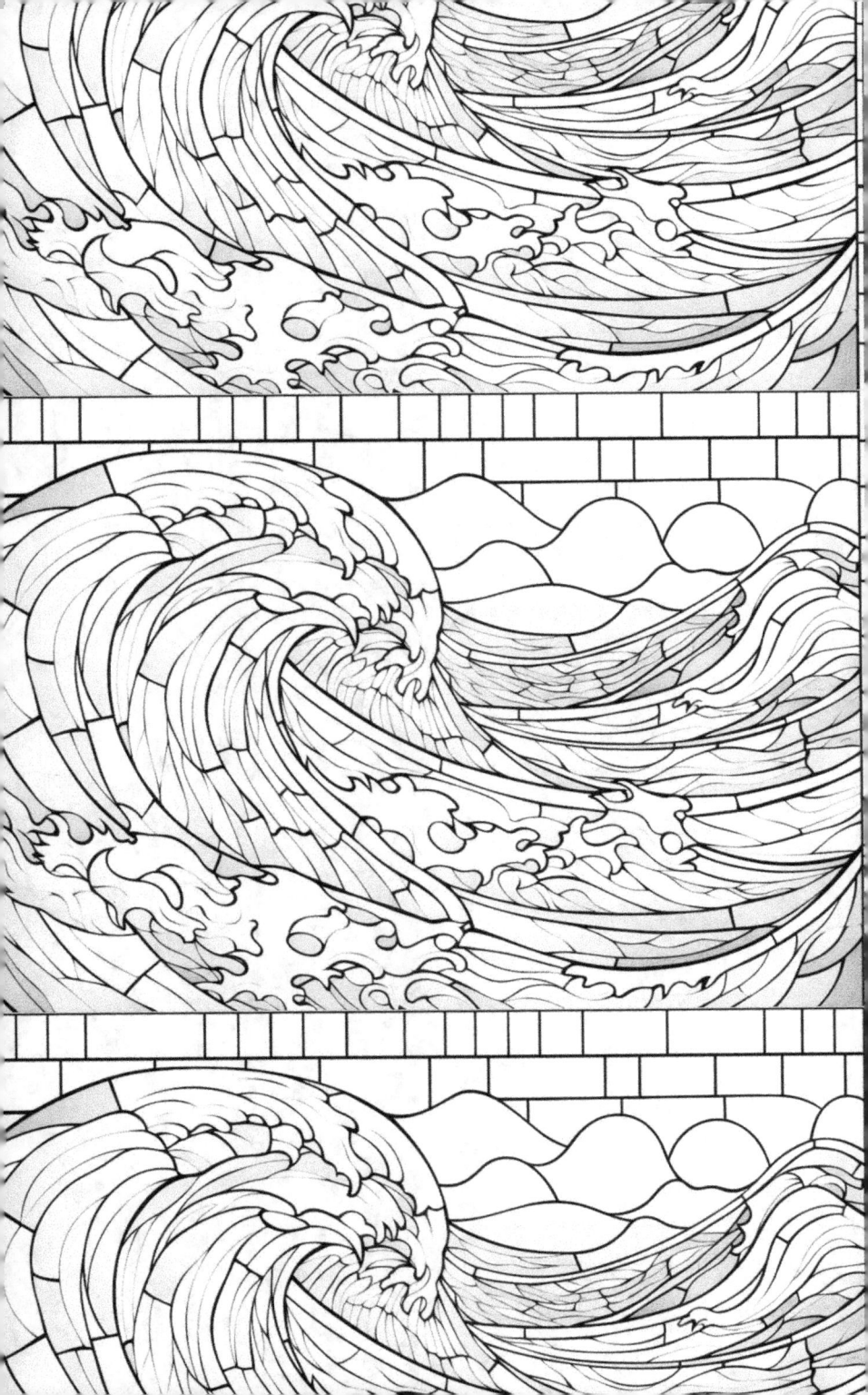

Bargaining

I know that bargaining with God isn't effective, but I still thought about it — still said, "Not him... and why not me?"

I suppose I bargain with myself as a way of life: after 5 workouts, you get cheesecake, or finish 50 pages, then you get a massage.

The bargaining stage is about making promises to yourself or a higher being, asking the universe for a chance to put things right. A bereaved person may seek reason where there is none, and may feel guilty about how they behaved, or carry blame.

What-if thoughts are edgy and intrusive during this stage as the answer to each what-if will only serve to intensify the presence of guilt and blame.

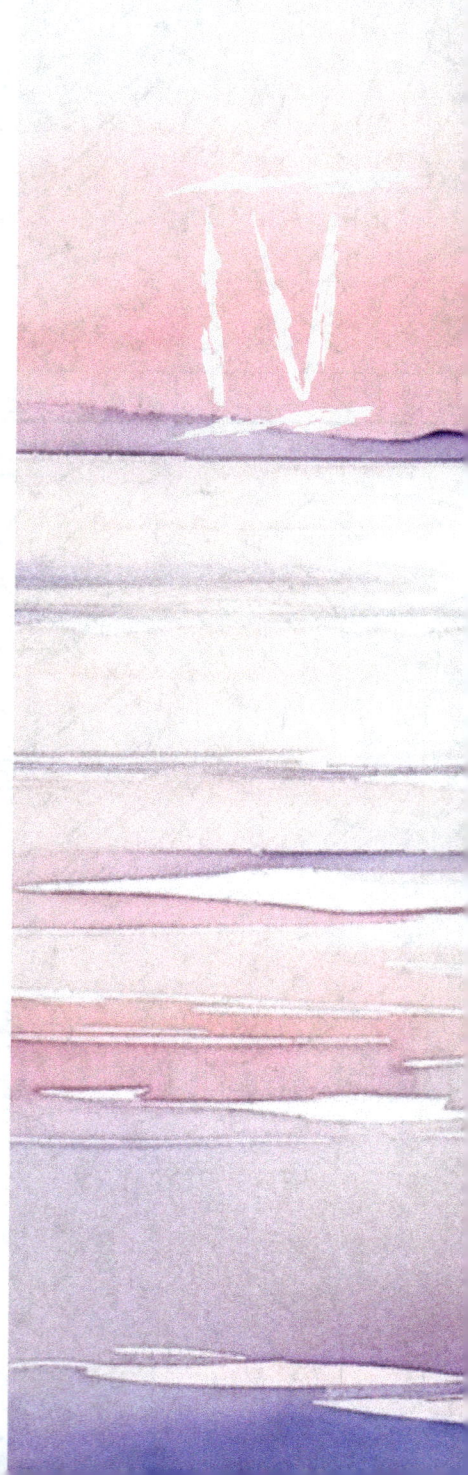

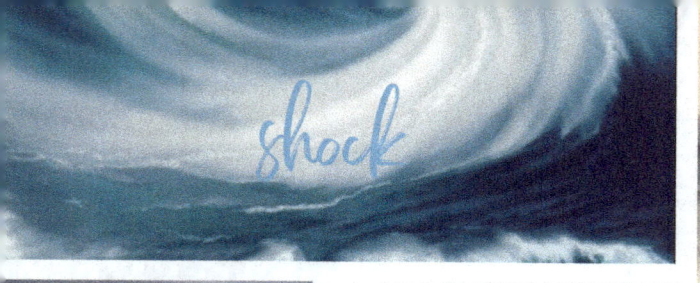
shock

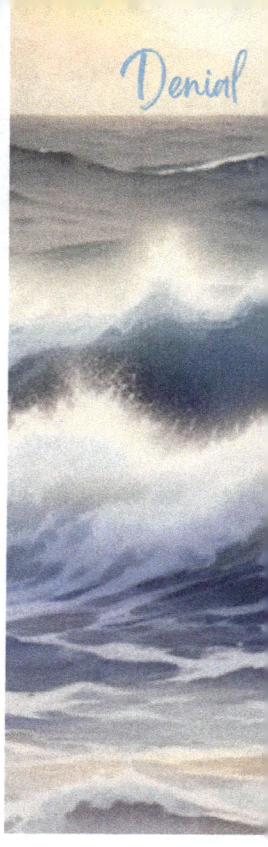
Denial

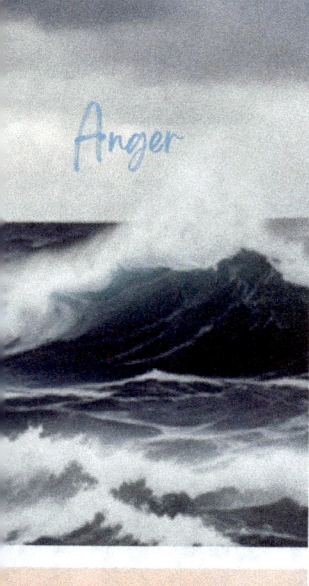
Anger

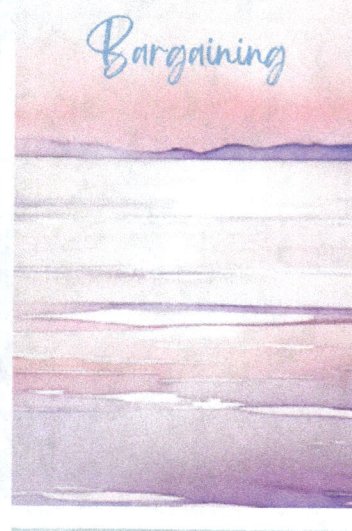
Bargaining

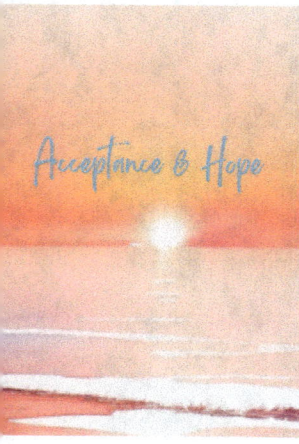
Acceptance & Hope

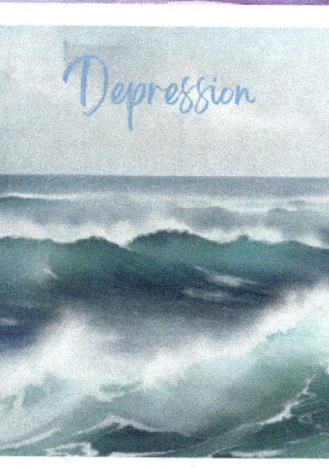
Depression

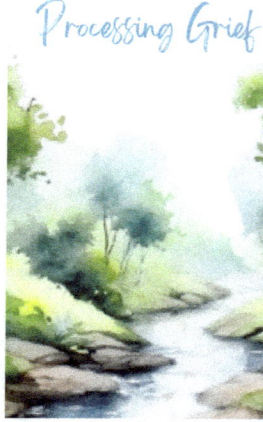
Processing Grief

Where Are You Today?

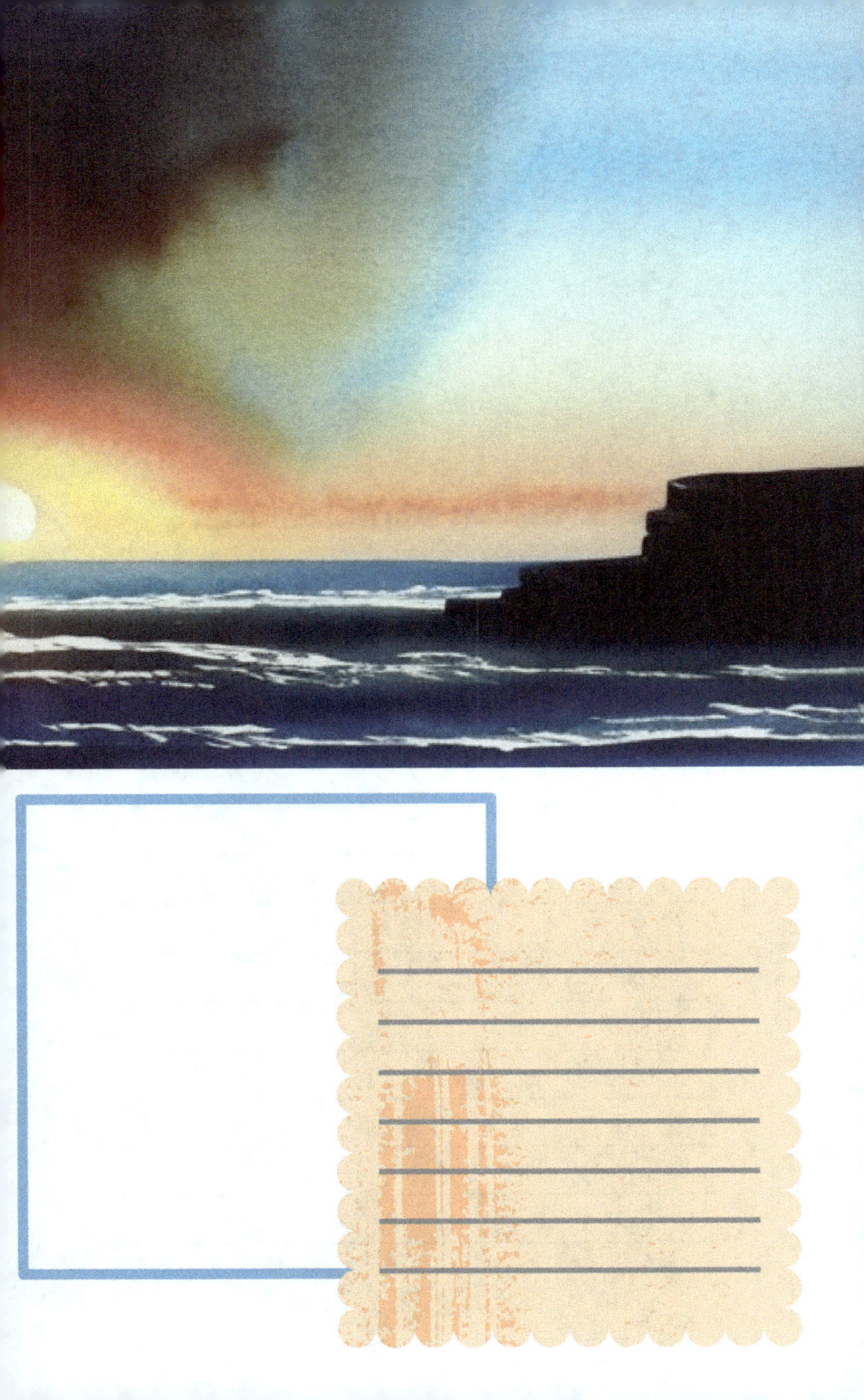

Check-In

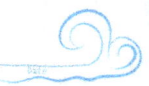

Remember to Be where you Are.
Reflect on your dominant
emotions and what's captivating
your mind? What is your
greatest need right now?

_____
_____
_____
_____
_____
_____
_____
_____
_____
_____
_____

Possible Prompts

If you have experienced guilt along your grief journey — write about your feelings.

What happened? Give yourself permission to tell your story and to navigate in the way you need to.

Express your grief outwardly — allow yourself to be where you are. Write about what you are suppressing?

Name your support systems and who you can confide in. Sharing is vital to healthy healing.

What daily routines can you continue or begin that will contribute to your overall health and wellness?

What is your greatest need at this moment?

Reflect and write about your nutrition and water intake. Our body needs to be healthy to heal. Are there any changes you want to make?

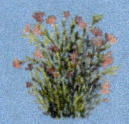

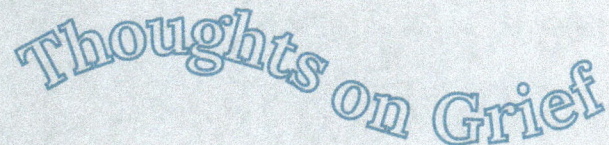

Two Years...

Its been two years my love and I still can't believe you're gone
So many reminders of you – my life is still singing your song
I feel the void of losing you as soon as I open my eyes each day
That's when I close my eyes again, and I begin to pray
Asking God to give me strength and to please show me the way
Because my life feels like a jungle and I'm lost, trying to find a way out
There are thorns and vines and snakes and sadly no one hears me when I shout
It's dark in here, thick and heavy and there's no end in sight.
But then, when I look up, somehow God always shows me the light.
I take one step at a time and trust in Him to keep me on solid ground
Although I'm sad and scared, greater faith is what I found.
I do believe that I will get out of here and one day my life will feel brand new
And instead I'll carry all my memories and love as special reminders of what I shared with you
The jungle will be replaced with the most beautiful beach I proclaim
Seagulls will sing your song my love and the waves will whisper your name

by Tonya Vann in loving memory of Steffon Vann
"Weeping to Winning: a Workbook for Widows"

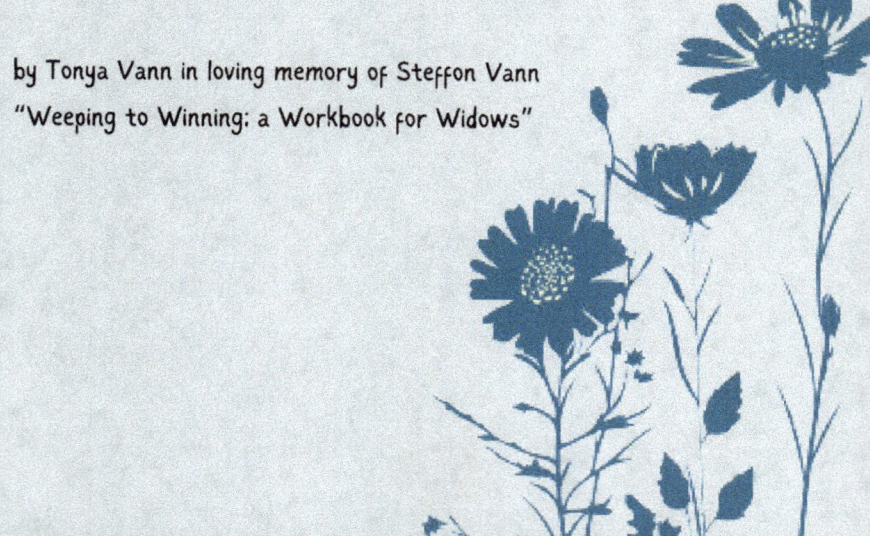

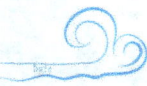

I can do all this through him
who gives me strength.

Philippians 4:13

_____

_____

_____

_____

_____

_____

_____

_____

_____

_____

_____

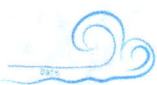

For God so loved the world that he gave
his one and only Son, that whoever
believes in him shall not perish but
have eternal life.

John 3:16

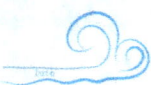

Self-Care Check

Exercise & Activities

How much
water did you
drink today?

What was the best
part of your day?

Who are you grateful
for? Who or what made
a difference in your day?

The Mighty Tear Collector

If I had to choose one scripture that offered me the greatest comfort when my head was beneath the water, it would be Psalm 56:8.

That our Lord keeps track of my sorrows and collects my tears always settles my aching heart. I am keenly aware that He walks with me, but Psalm 56:8 reminds me how deeply He cares and that His compassion is unmatched. I am reminded of the aches and agony when one of my sons suffer... and how I long to comfort and heal. I am reminded that our Father desires nothing less for me. I am reminded that I am loved.

> You keep track of all my sorrows. You have collected all my tears in your bottle. You have recorded each one in your book.
>
> Psalm 56:8
> NLT

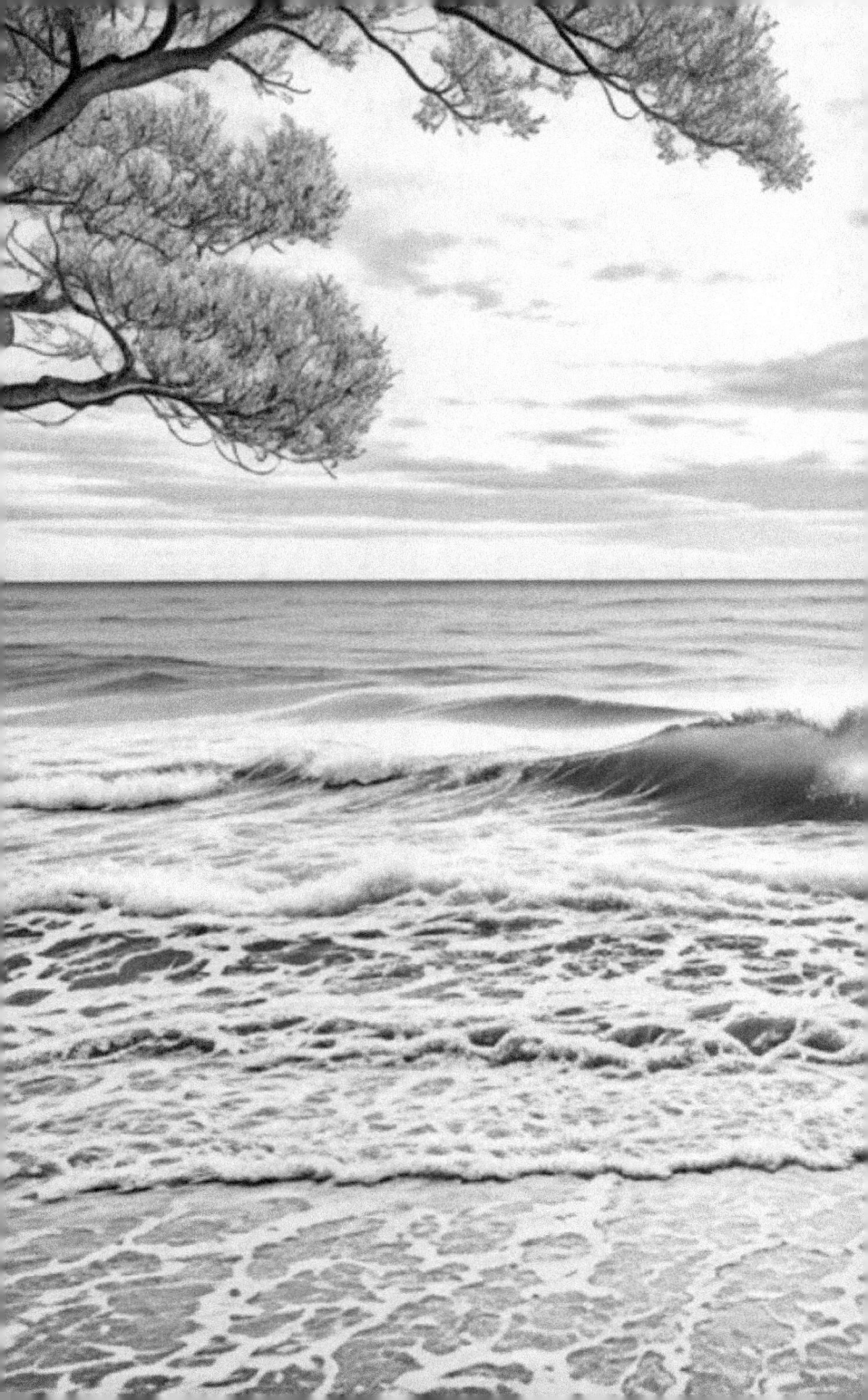

Depression

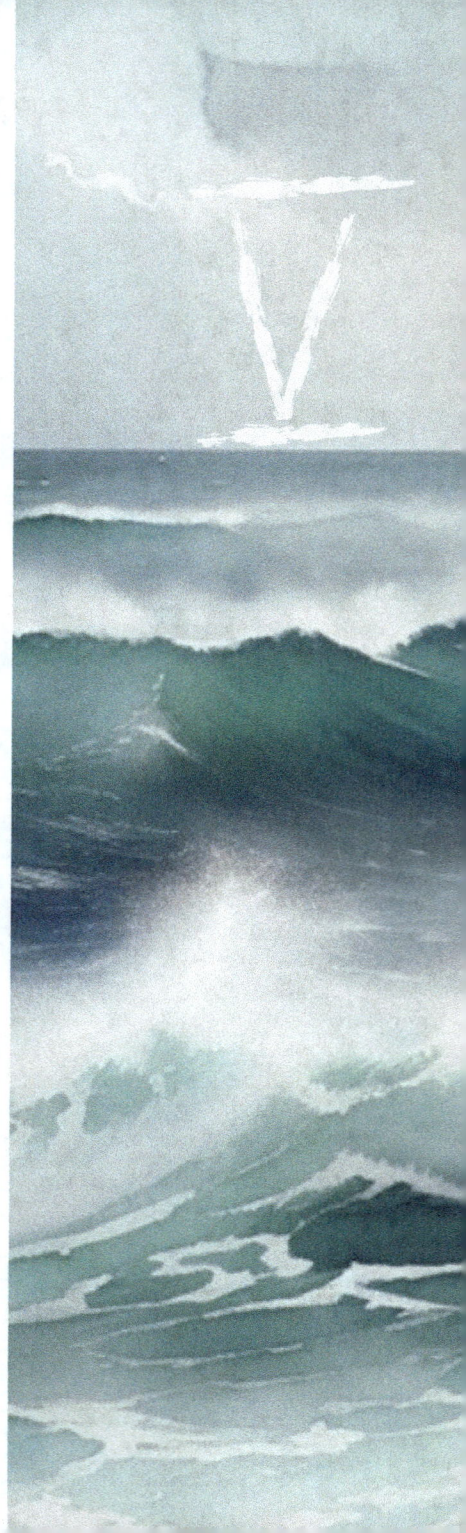

The hopelessness was overwhelming. I dreaded facing my parents and seeing their hurt. I couldn't see the sunshine or flowers or any of the usual things that brought me joy. My family was around, but I never felt this kind of pure loneliness — I wanted to sleep until everything passed.

This was the way my depression moved. Lack of energy, drive, and purpose topped with fear defined this season.
I don't think I was suicidal, but it was most definitely a dark, cold, and isolating space, without an EXIT sign. It is SO important that you reach out for help and share with your inner circle how you are feeling.

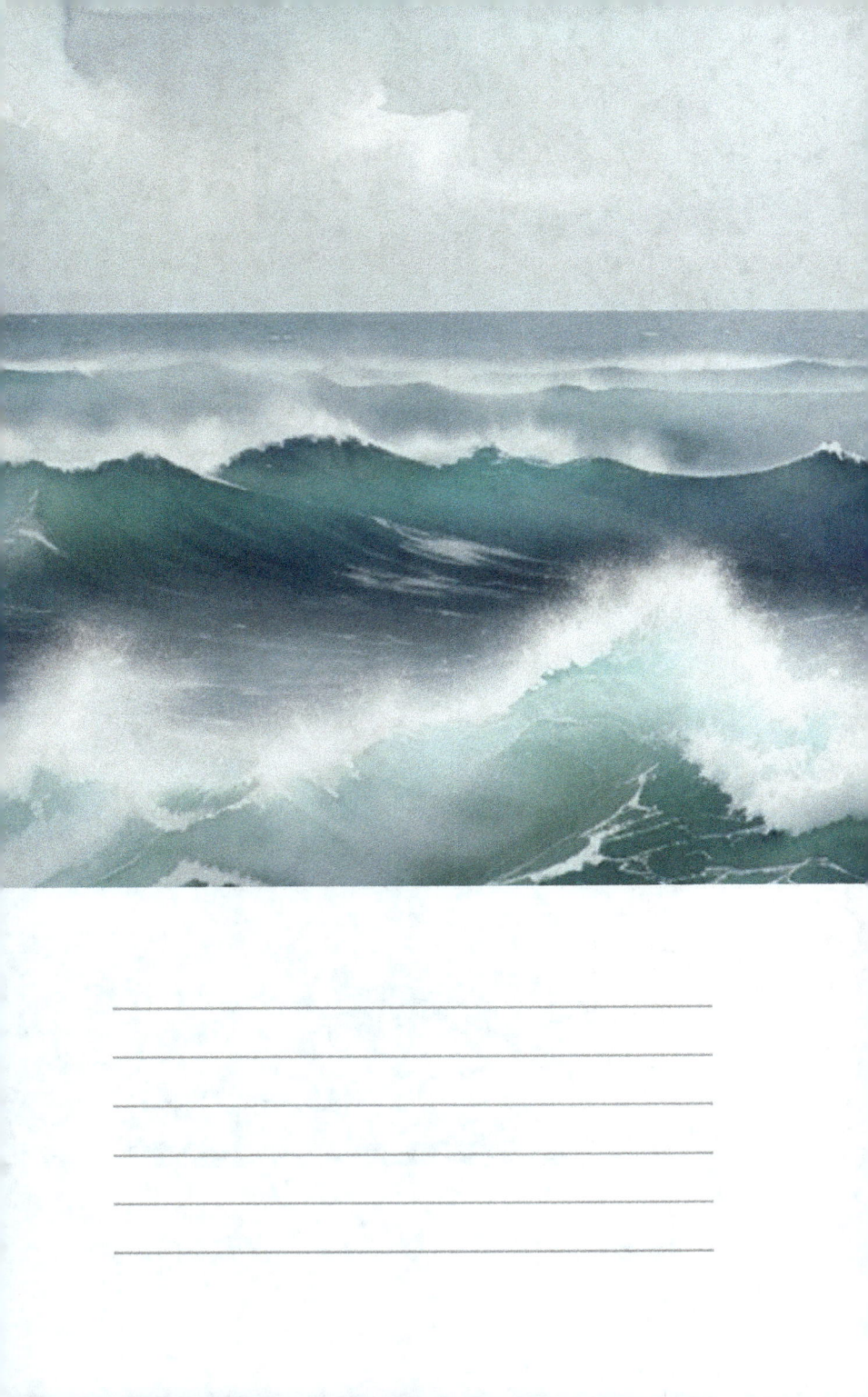

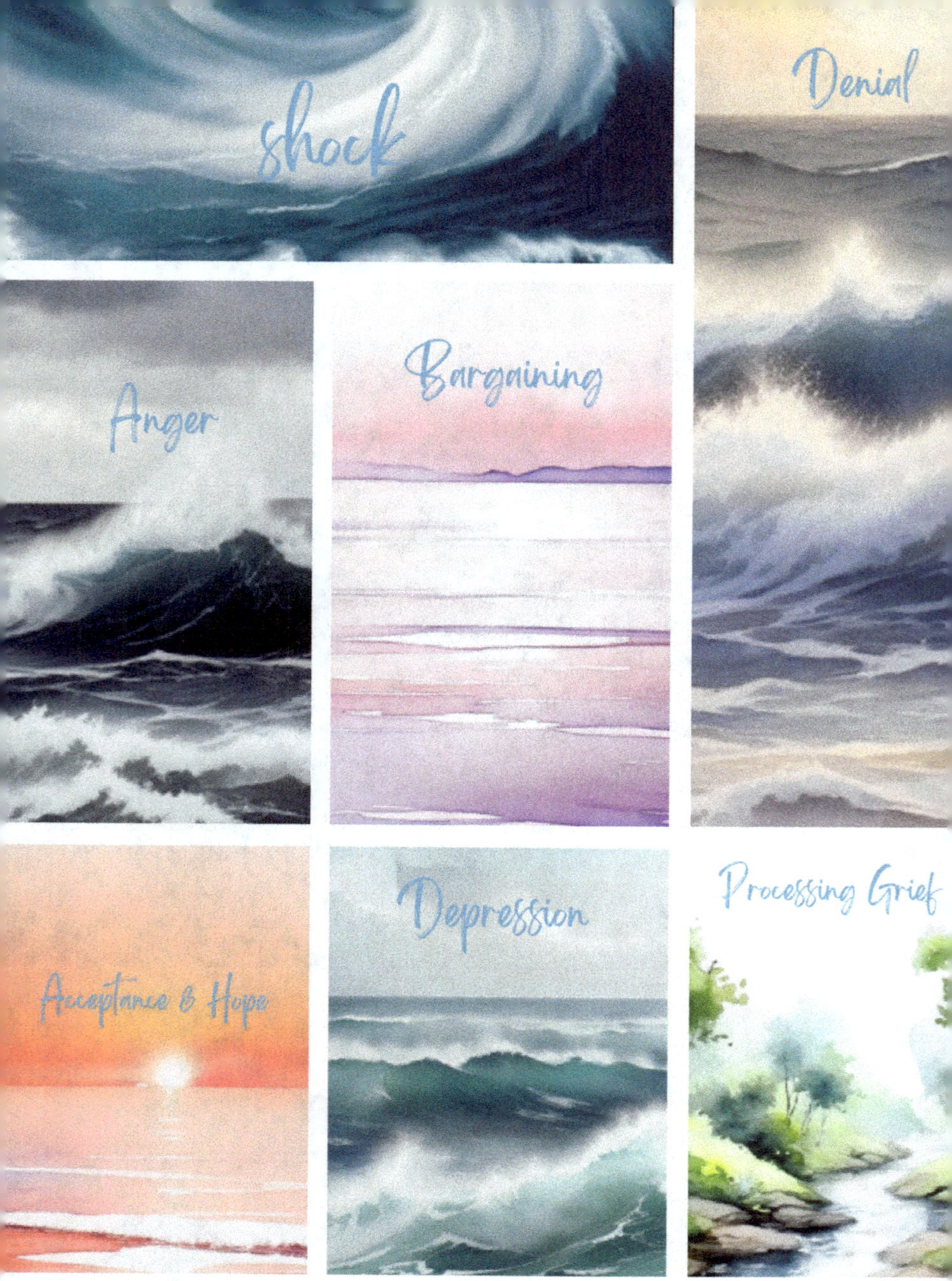

Shock

Denial

Anger

Bargaining

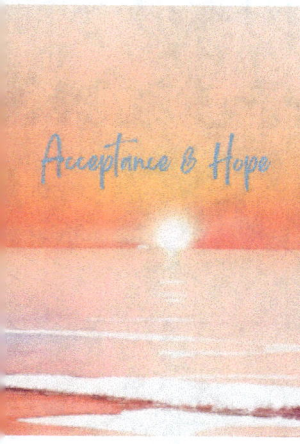

Depression

Acceptance & Hope

Processing Grief

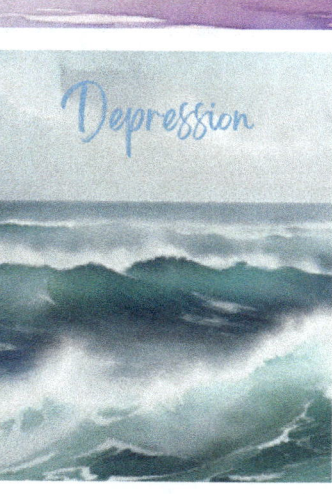

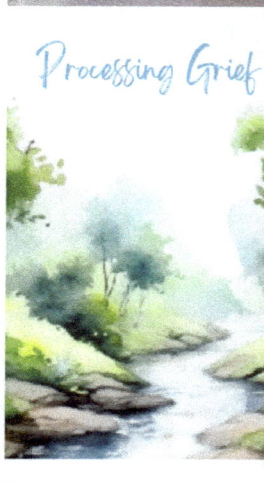

Where Are You Today?

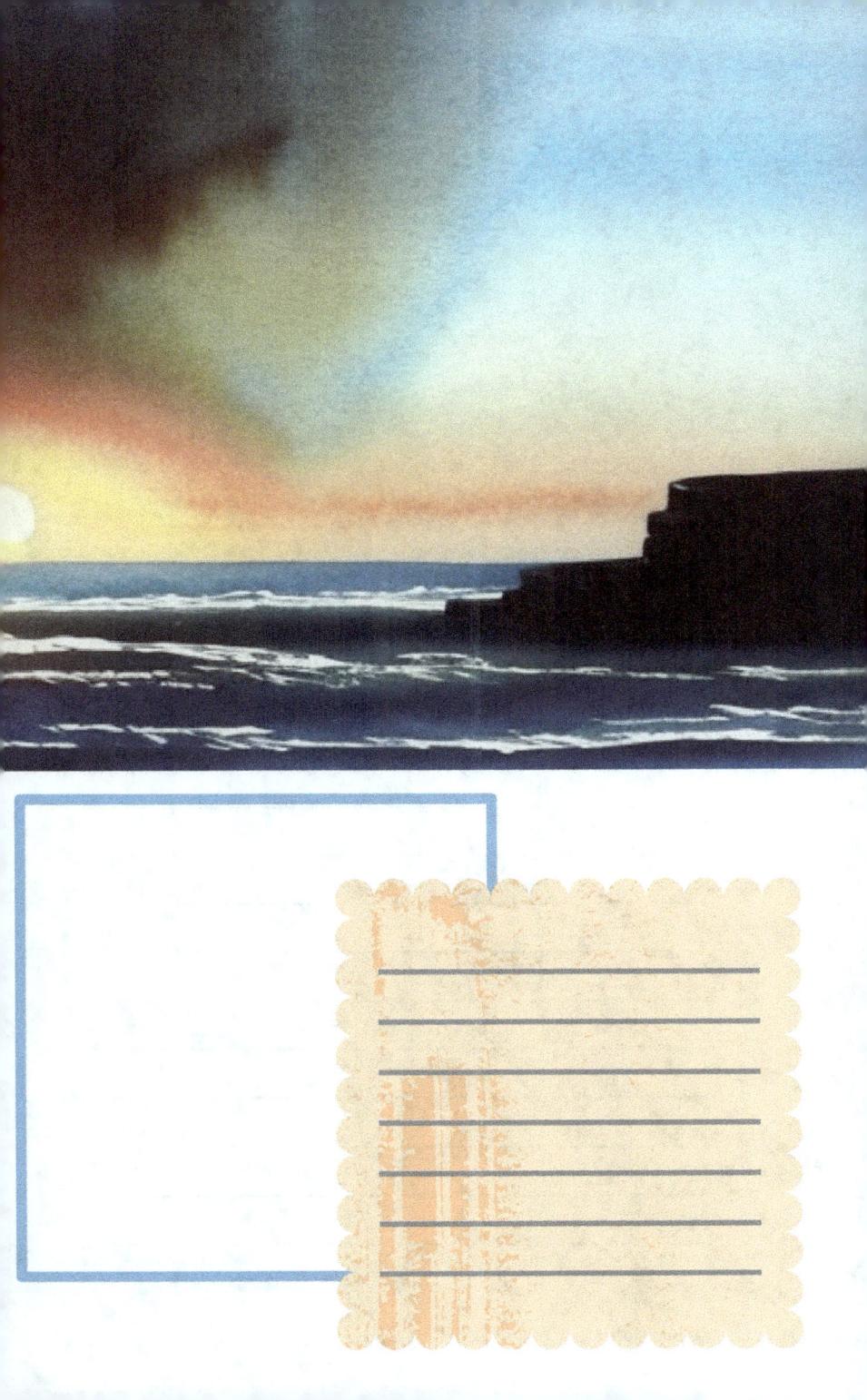

Check-In

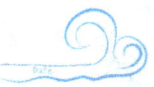

It's a good time to check-in on You. Reflect on your dominant emotions and what's captivating your thoughts? What is your greatest need right now?

_____

_____

_____

_____

_____

_____

_____

_____

_____

_____

_____

Possible Prompts

Describe how depression manifests in your body — where do you feel it?

Consider all that you have overcome. Write a letter to yourself as a reminder of your strength and resilience.

Have something to look forward to. What plans can you make (a vacation, spa day, girls night)?

Are there times of the year that are more difficult than others?

Write about a happy memory?

What false statements does your inner critic make? Explain why they are wrong.

Gratitude is deeply healing — write a list of things you are grateful for today.

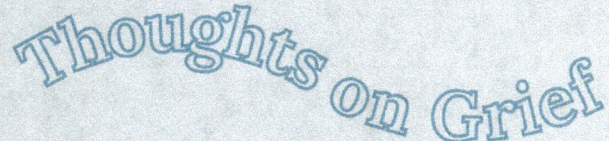

Thoughts on Grief

Nicola Dalbenzio reminds us that...

Stepping out in faith builds faith.
Grief is different.
Jesus weeps with us, as he did over
Lazarus and for those who wept for
Lazarus. He grieves with us and for
us.

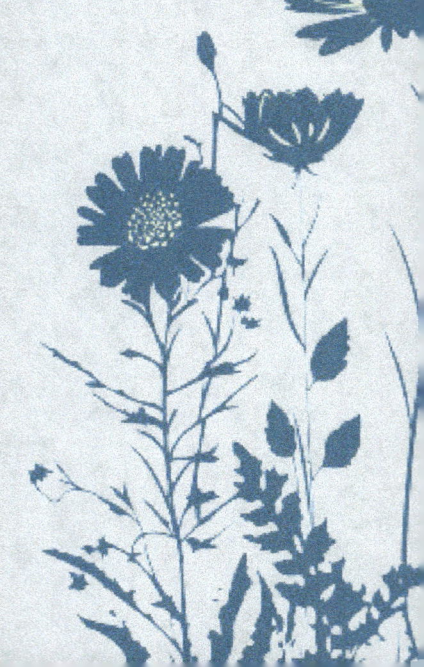

Jesus wept.

JOHN 11:35

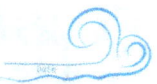

He says, "Be still, and know that I am God;
I will be exalted among the nations,
I will be exalted in the earth."

Psalm 46:10

_____
_____
_____
_____
_____
_____
_____
_____
_____
_____
_____

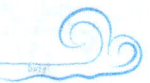

The LORD is close to the
brokenhearted and saves those who
are crushed in spirit.

Psalm 34:18

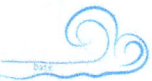

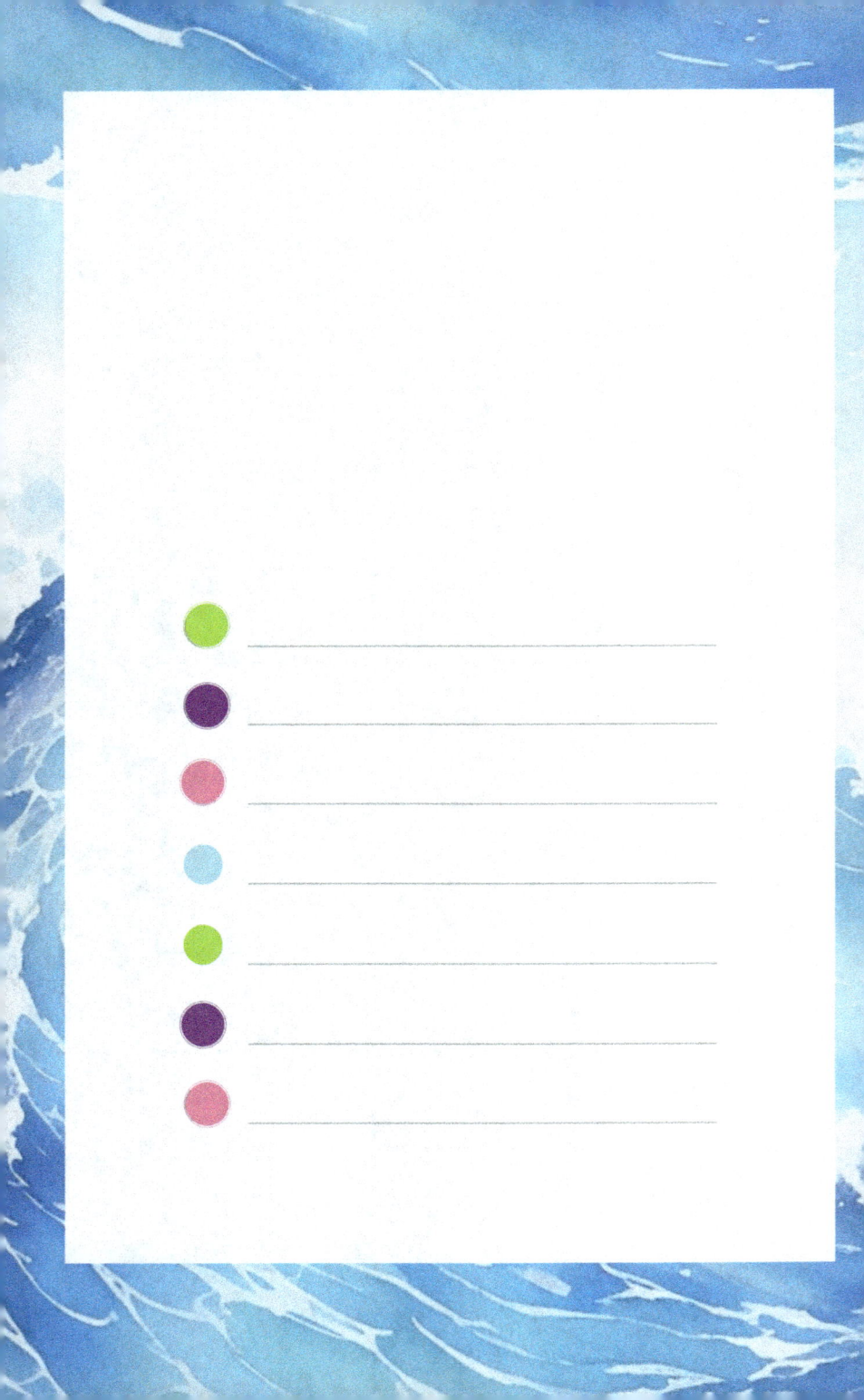

Self-Care Check

Exercise & Activities

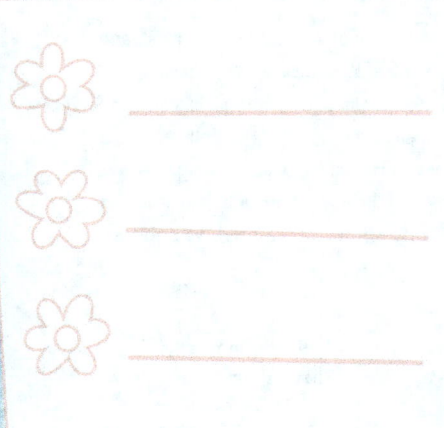

How much water did you drink today?

What was the best part of your day?

Who are you grateful for? Who or what made a difference in your day?

The Healing Power of Music

Gene Beresin says in, "The Power of Music: to Feel, Heal, and Connect, that, "Music is the best studied of art therapy and helps to lower anxiety, depression, trauma, psychosis and stress. Important components of music therapy are the meaning of lyrics, improvisational music playing, active listening, and songwriting." I hold writing and journaling in the same regard — but regardless of the form you choose, art is a powlerful elixir.

As a girl, I used to sit on the floor and write down the lyrics of my favorite songs. Imagine doing this with a portable cassette player... stop, rewind, play, stop, rewind, play. I didn't always get the lyrics right, but I loved the process. By college, I had stacks of 'Song-Books'. What was I really doing? I was searching for a deeper meaning hidden in the lyrics... perhaps revealed only to the seekers. I was healing.

Breathe in breathe out
That's all that I can do now
Hold on somehow
My world has come crashing down

And I cannot understand
How this could be your heart
Still I'm lifting trembling hands
Help me trust in who you are

You are my God
Here in the darkness in the night
You have never left my side
You are my God

Even when I can't see your face
I know I'm held in your embrace
You are my God

"You Are My God"
Recorded by Nicol Sponberg

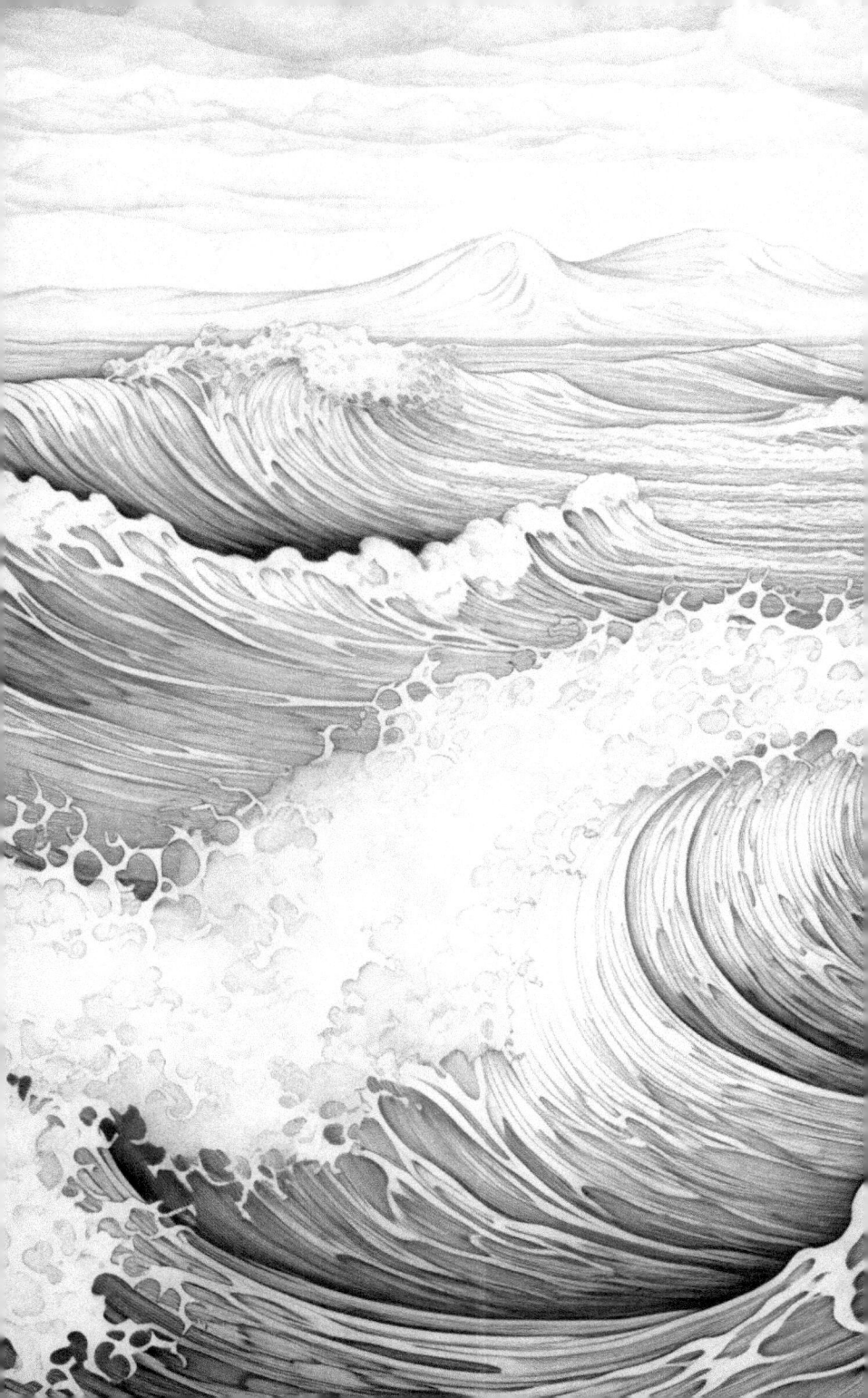

Acceptance & Hope

Acceptance & Hope
was initially the
stage I longed for,
but it turned out to
be more of the same.
You see, stage seven
is Processing.
So Acceptance & Hope
is in-between
Depression &
Processing – and for
some it feels like
both.

Confusion could ensue
as you may
experience all of the
emotions again (from
day to day or moment
to moment).

Be deliberate & be
patient with yourself.
Allow yourself to Be
where you Are.

There is Hope within
Self-Acceptance.

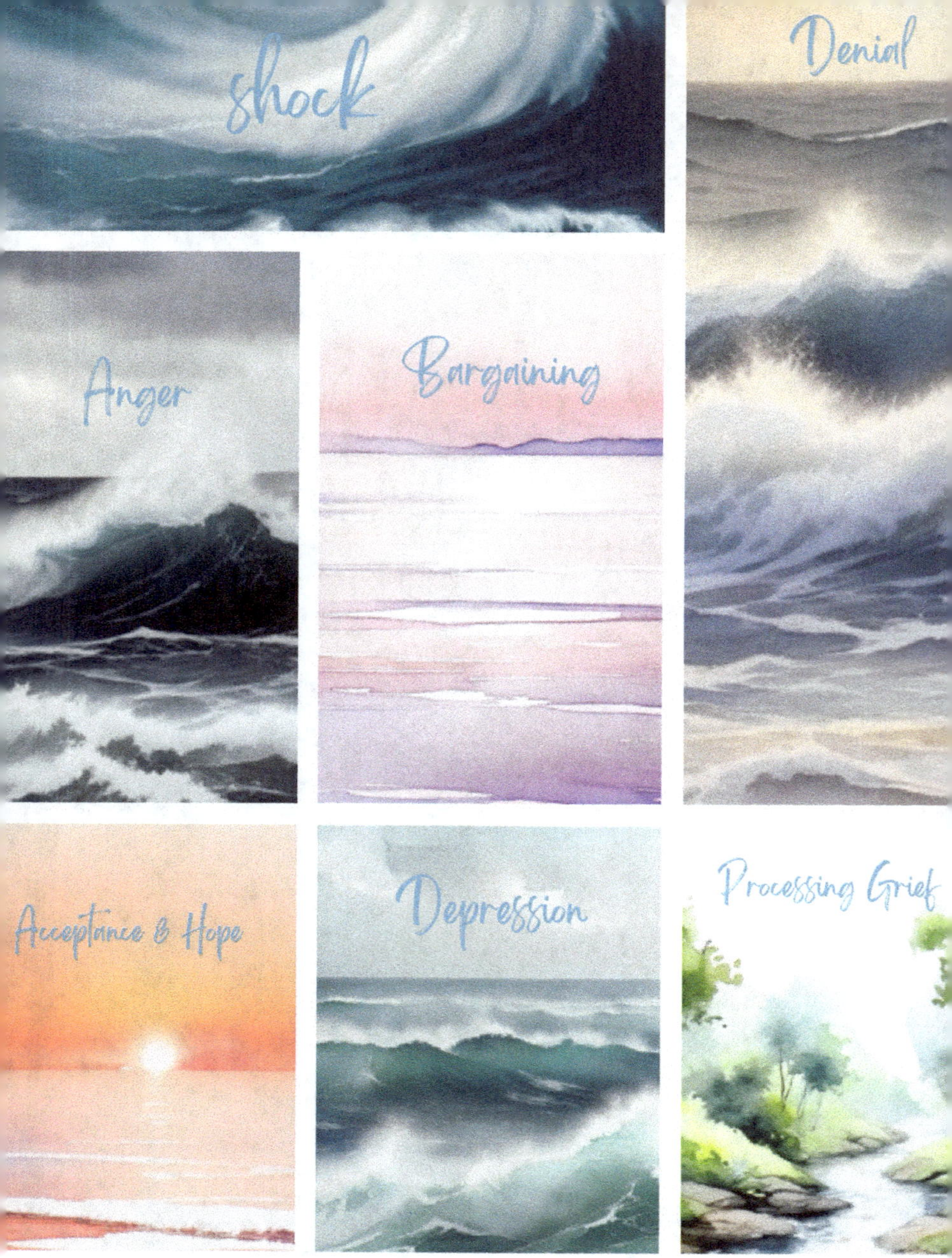

shock

Denial

Anger

Bargaining

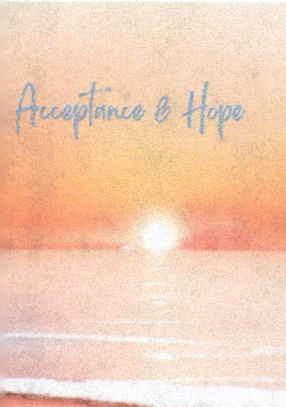

Acceptance & Hope

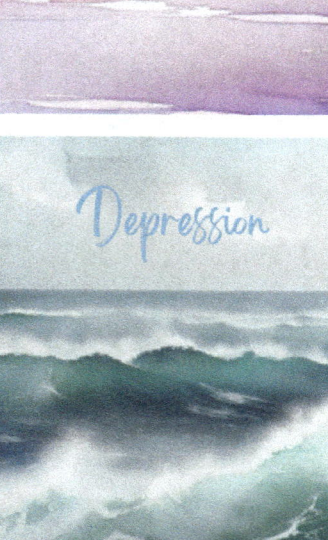

Depression

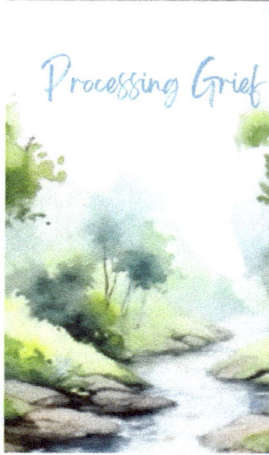

Processing Grief

Where Are You Today?

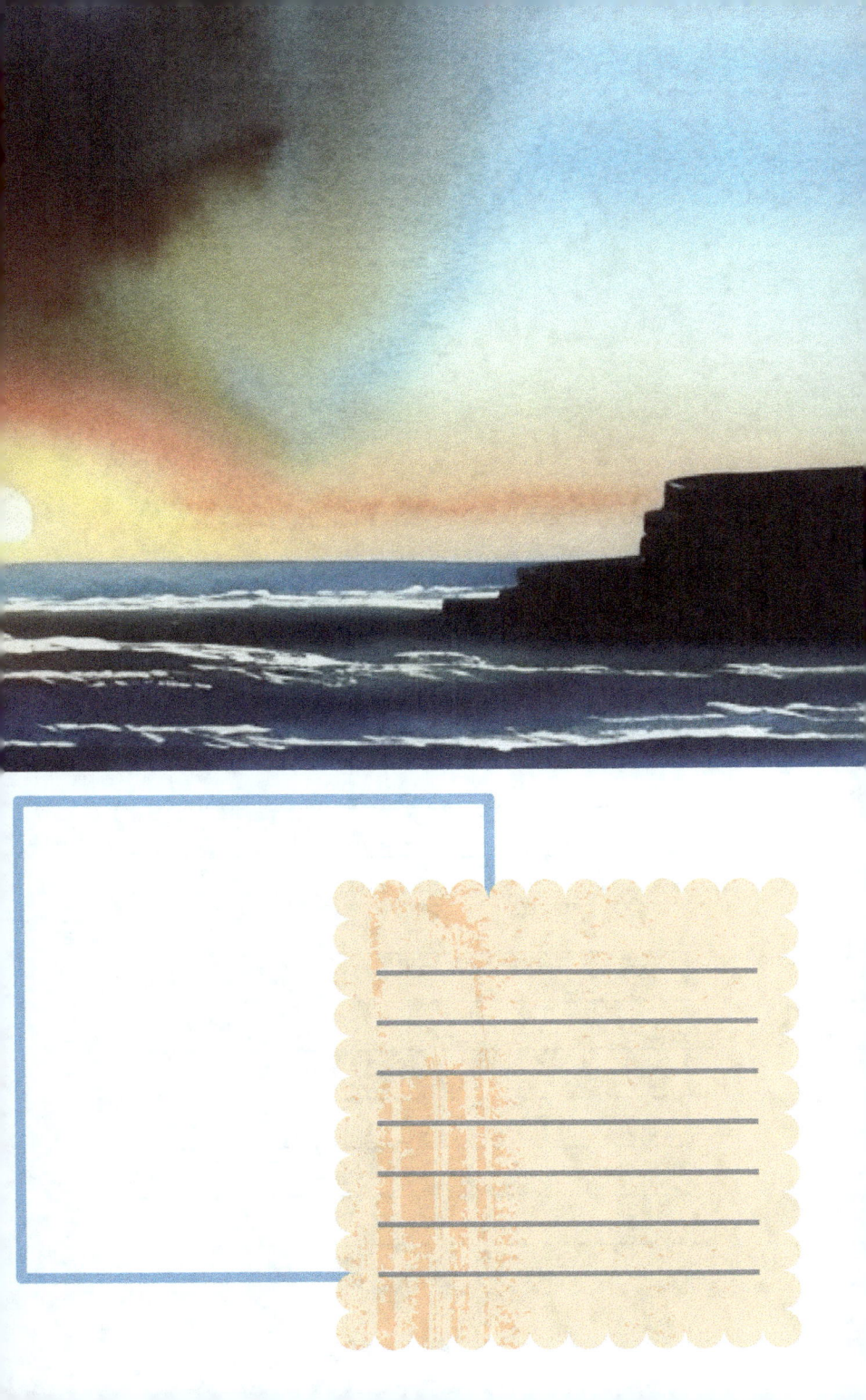

Check-In

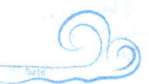

Remember to Be where you Are. Reflect on your dominant emotions and what's captivating your mind? What is your greatest need right now?

_____

_____

_____

_____

_____

_____

_____

_____

_____

_____

Prompts & Activities to Express Your Heart Creatively

What tree or flower represents cherished memories?

💜 Consider planting a remembrance tree or shrub

💜 Consider planting special flowers

Perusing through old photos can be nostalgic and healing in time.

💜 Consider creating a digital photo album

💜 Consider a scrapbook or cookbook

What thoughts and feelings do you most want to release?

💜 Consider a Healing, Self-Growth or Self-Care Journal

💜 Try writing your feelings as a poem, song, or letter

What is an art or craft you have always wanted to learn?

💜 Consider looking for local beginning classes (salsa, ballroom dance, box gardens, or guitar lessons)

💜 Consider asking someone you know to teach you something they are good at (a green-thumb, plant-based meals, pickle-ball)

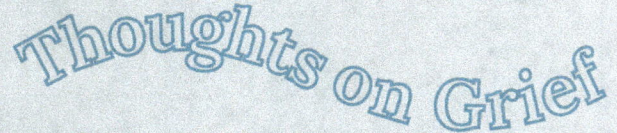

Thoughts on Grief

Finding Your Way Through the Darkness

by Karen Smith

Finding a way to begin to deal with grief proved more challenging than I could have imagined. Some moments were (and continue to be) filled with absolute despair and led me to cry endlessly. I often felt that I was in the midst of a world filled with darkness from which I could not see any hope of escape. I reached depths that made me wish I was the one who died... I wanted to join him above. Going on felt hopeless, but for some unknown reason I continued to try.

I'm not sure why, but I knew he would want me to be strong and to never ever consider death an alternative for myself. I knew that would completely disappoint him... he expects more of us regardless of how deeply we mourn his loss. Nevertheless, each day when I opened my eyes and then closed them again at night, I dreaded and feared the cold and bitter hours to come.

Then somewhat suddenly, I would be filled with some of the most wonderful memories: memories of my son who I loved beyond life itself... seemingly endless tears would change before my eyes and become exquisite visions of laughter and joy and fun. They are visions I tried desperately to sustain, but which inevitably were fleeting, and I would find myself once again immersed in deep unrelenting sadness.

Day after day, night after night, the months passed and then the years and this repetitive cycle only made the loss more and more unbearable. I began to wonder what the future could possibly hold for me now following the devastating reality I knew I must somehow face.

Finally, just as I thought I had given up hope, after endless hours of searching and prayer, my soul was lifted back into the world where I had been blessed to know true beauty and strength... the world before death and grief had consumed me.

Yes, through unexpected grace, the spirit can lift us up and carry us back into the place where life's joys and blessings are present. Believe me, it can happen. It is perhaps through kindnesses given and moments shared or as it was for me, through the realizations of just how very much I still had in this world.

As I consider what or who lifted me, I realized it was my wonderful family. While there were days I felt like I was failing everyone I loved, my husband stepped in and filled the gaps. My partner and wonderful spouse was (and is) absolutely unbelievable in every way. I thank our Lord for the blessing of a kind and giving husband.

Our two grandsons have been remarkable, each in their individual ways. Our youngest with his curiosity, resilience, and great sense of adventure and our oldest with his incredible faith and wisdom beyond his years. Unexpectedly, our oldest asked to come and live with us for a time. It was a great surprise that enabled us to spend time with him we had not had since he was a child. What an opportunity for us to get to know him as a young man. Somehow, he has managed to reach out through his own grief over the loss of his uncle and touch my heart and soul as one much older than his years would indicate. He has spent untold hours sharing his beliefs and faith with me. How blessed I have been to see God through the eyes of this young Christian visionary; he truly enriches my spirit... getting me more centered with my faith and our Lord.

It is most unusual to be blessed with a son-in-law who is truly a good man, a good husband, and a great father, but to find all of this in a package that also includes a considerate and thoughtful man is quite unbelievable. But to add these characteristics to any that also include those of a spiritual nature, you might think nearly impossible to find but, in this case, it is actually the reality... a blessed man of God leads this family through its highs and lows, making grieving more bearable to transcend.

And finally, and again most remarkably, there is our daughter. Our son's little sister. After all the endless hours of searching for answers, asking for help, looking for resources, seeking renewed faith, and turning to our Lord in prayer, my greatest source of strength became clearly evident right before my eyes. It was just as it had always been throughout their lives, his little sister... Baby Girl was there for him and now for me.

It really should have been no surprise that she was there for the rest of our family. She is the beacon flashing before our downcast eyes, lighting our way through the darkest of nights. How could I have struggled so long failing to see the precious gift God had put before me? My other child...

It is when we can finally clear our eyes, our hearts, and our minds, that we will recognize the blessings we have had all along... The gifts of those right beside us each day magically who reach out to us knowing just what to do or say. While the pain may continue to periodically rise from deep within, my prayer for each of us who must learn the name of grief is that, in time, you too will connect with your special ones who will bring you immeasurable relief and allow all the love you can imagine living in you once again.

After all, it is through the love we are given and give in return that we become inspired and renewed and ultimately, will find the path we need to move out of darkness into the light.

For me, the love and support of my family was the key to surviving. I learned that grief is not a journey we can or should walk alone.

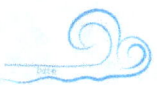

Brothers, we do not want you to be ignorant about those who fall asleep, or to grieve like the rest of men, who have no hope. 14 We believe that Jesus died and rose again and so we believe that God will bring with Jesus those who have fallen asleep in him.

1 Thessalonians 4:13-14

And we know that in all things God
works for the good of those who
love him, who have been called
according to his purpose.

Romans 8:28

_____

_____

_____

_____

_____

_____

_____

_____

_____

_____

Finding the Words

Regardless of my current stage of grief or emotional extremes, I have consistently found joy when I take a fond memory and use it to create something tangible that captures my feelings.
I've written, painted, planted...
Drawn, sewed, sang...
(I didn't say well!)

It took me awhile to find my words and figure out what exactly I want to say, but I've always felt better after taking the time to express myself creatively.

I imagine Alicia Keyes singing Dance, Dance, Dance.

Is there a song or poem in you that needs to make it to the page?

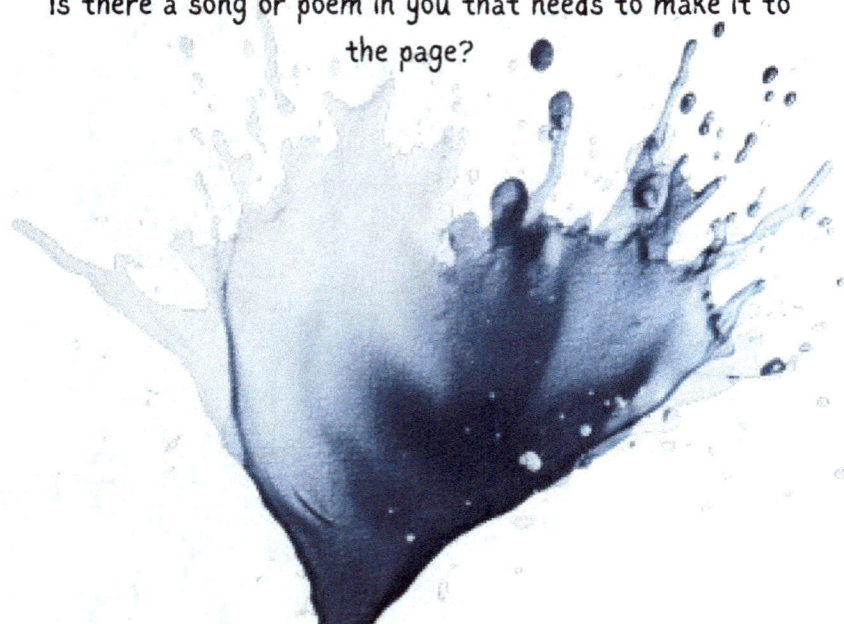

Dance, Dance, Dance
for James-Kious Kelly

You were there from the start,
always
Always there to pick up the pieces
And dry my eyes

You'd say,
"It's alright, Babygirl, don't you cry
Stand back up – learn to fight
This world ain't kind, you gotta take
it by the reigns
Be you, be true...
Don't live in shame

I say...
Dance, dance, dance
Dance down the street
Just as you please
The world is your stage
Don't live on your knees

Yeah...
Dance, dance, dance
Find the beat of your drum
Dance, dance, dance
Never accept no."

Brother, I need you still
But you're not here
No cardinals or photos make you feel
near
Brother, so much I'd tell
Could we meet in a dream
I'll go anywhere to see you...
We don't have to talk, I just want to
see you
And hear you say...

It's alright, Babygirl, don't you cry
You gotta stand back up – learn to
fight
This world ain't kind, you gotta take
it by the reigns
Be you, be true...
Don't live in shame

Life is bitter without you
Your essence is so sweet
I cry out sometimes
But mostly I dance
You gave so much
Because of you, I get another chance

I'm gonna do like you told me...

Yeah...

Dance, dance, dance
Dance down the street
Just as I please
The world is my stage
I won't live on my knees

I'm gonna
Dance, dance, dance
Just as I please.

Yeah...

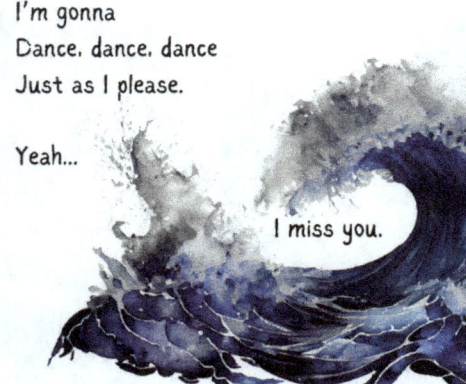

I miss you.

Self-Care Check

Exercise & Activities

How much water did you drink today?

What was the best part of your day?

Who are you grateful for? Who or what made a difference in your day?

The impact grief has on a person creeps into every aspect of your life. Know this and be understanding and kind to yourself, knowing that it is normal to not feel like yourself. In the midst of grief it feels as if you are lost and don't have the capacity to know it will get better. It is easy to forget or to not know that your mind and body are resilient beyond expectation and that you will not always be in the place you find yourself in during the storm of grief.

~ Omar Zaheer

I watched this young man routinely go away to pray in-between his remarkable stories about about vet life and exotic birds. It took no time at all for me to fall in love with his heart.

On the shore of a distant Fijian island, we shared about our loss, saying goodbye, and what drives us to live fully and without regret. Omar is one of the lasting gifts of my Survivor 42 experience.

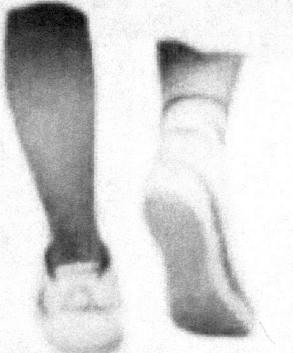

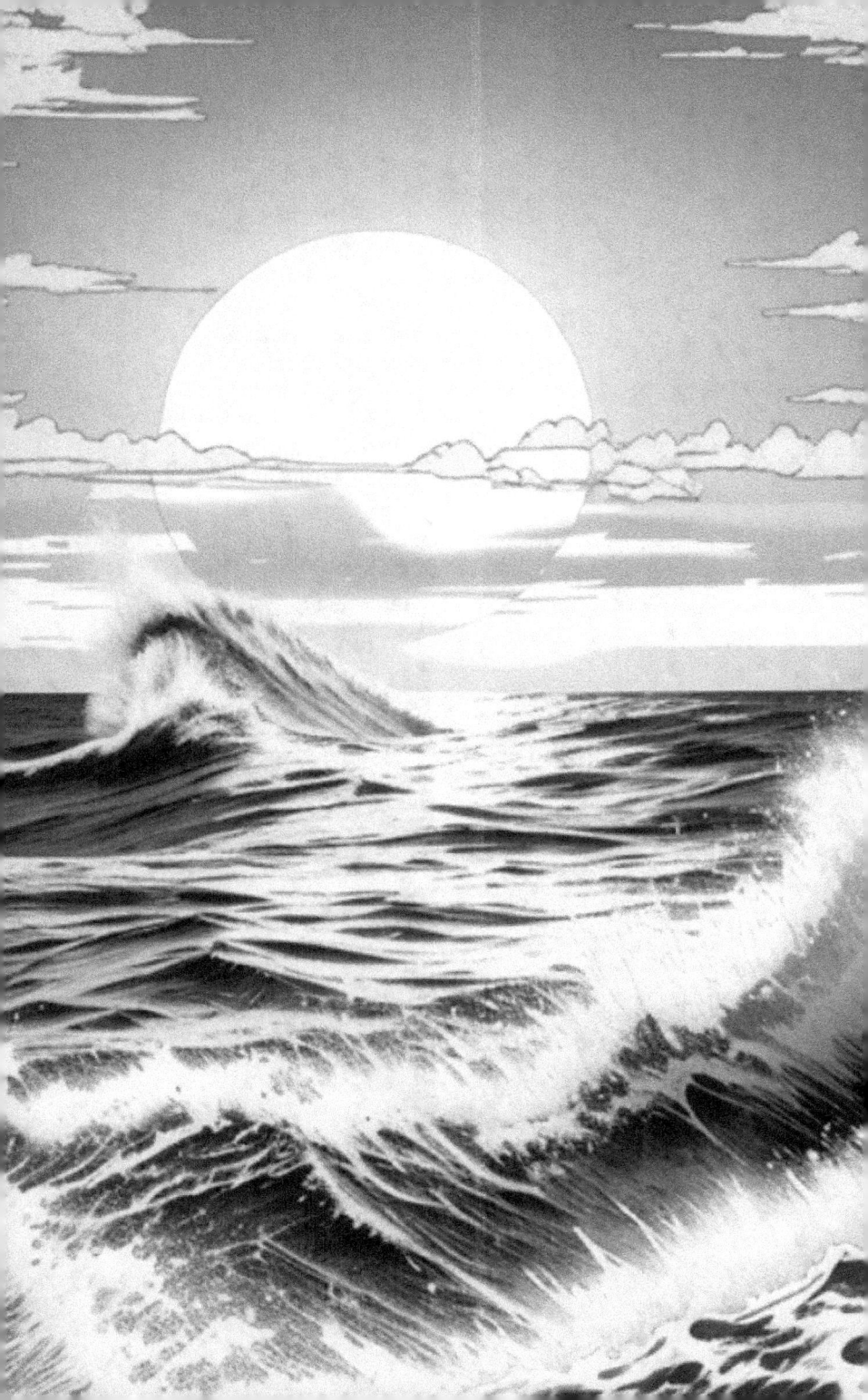

Processing Grief

Unlike the other stages, processing is something you want to experience. Perhaps unpleasant, but necessary. The alternative to processing... well, is not processing. This would most likely mean remaining in denial.

Healing (not forgetting) is on the other side of processing. Processing may be the most unique and individualized stage.

Tips for processing include: expressing your grief artistically, attending grief support groups, taking care of your self physically (rest, nutrition, and activity).

Being mindful of where you are will help in knowing when you are ready to process. We can't process while we are in shock, or anger, or bargaining for that matter.
Allow yourself to Be Where You Are... but be mindful of where you want to go.

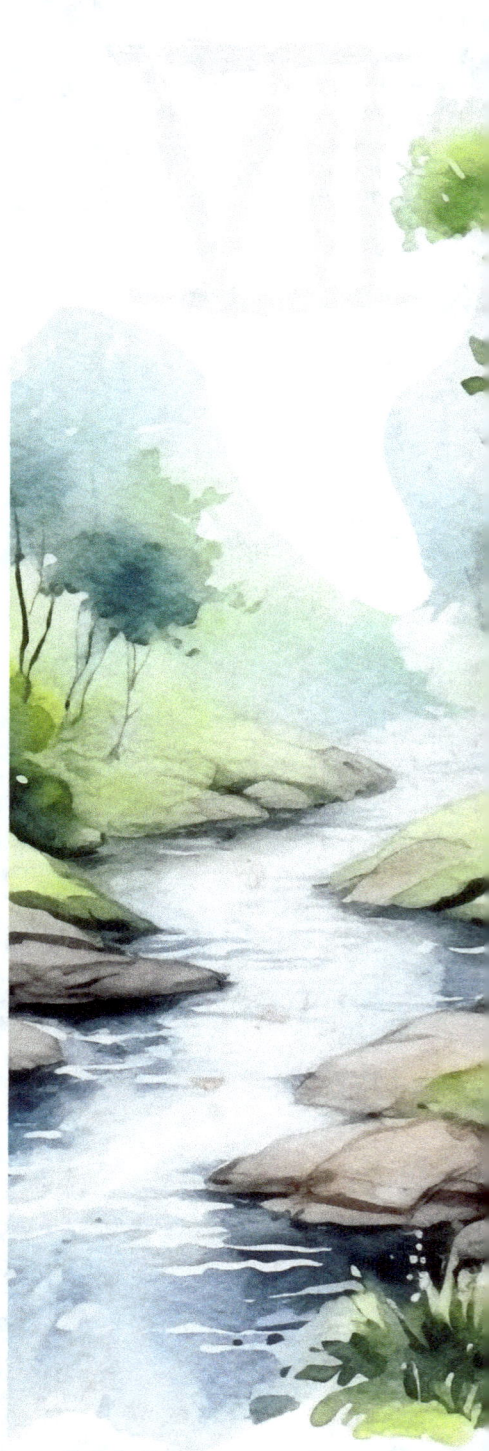

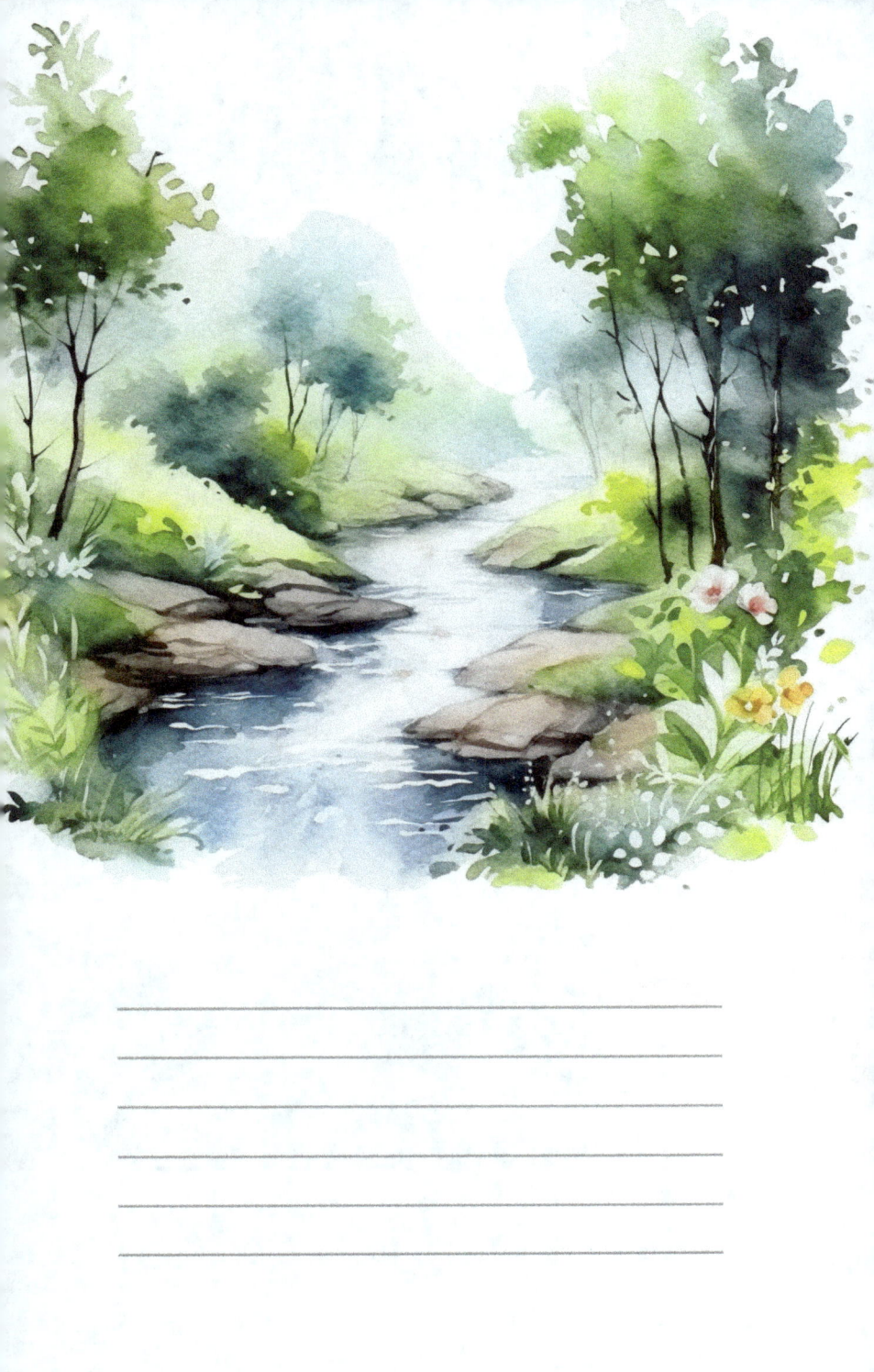

_____

_____

_____

_____

_____

_____

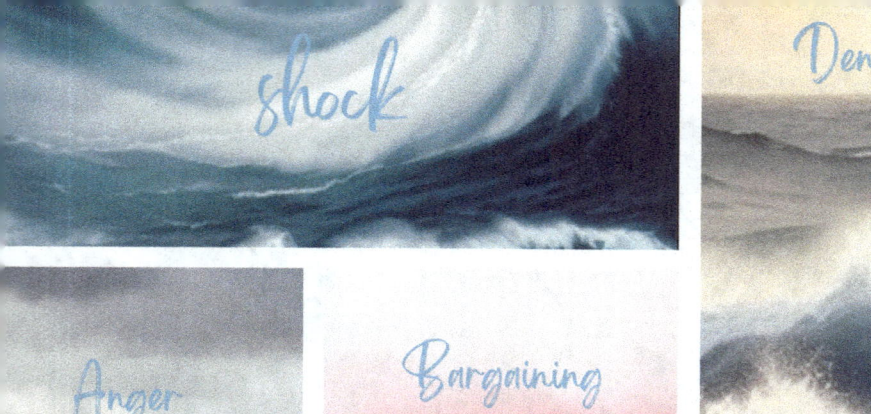

Shock

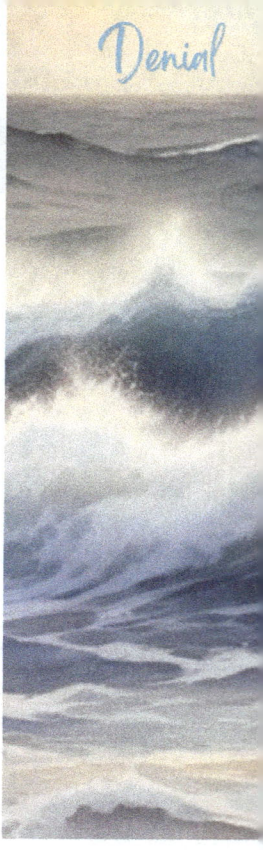

Denial

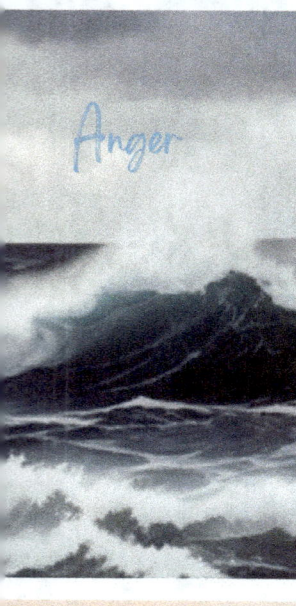

Anger

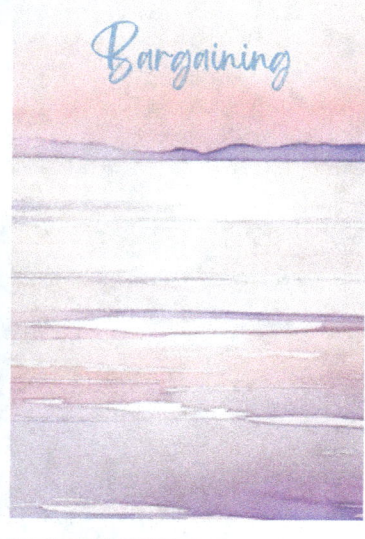

Bargaining

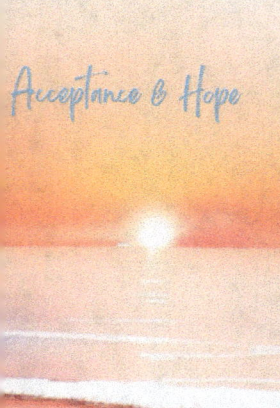

Acceptance & Hope

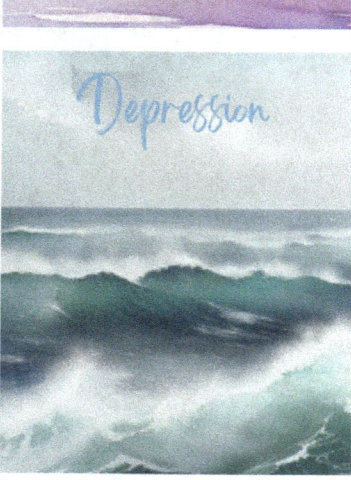

Depression

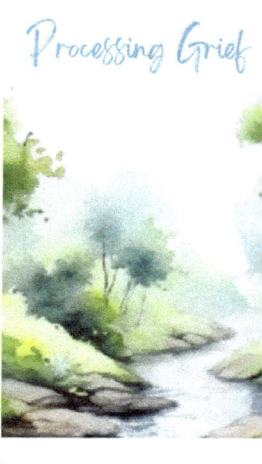

Processing Grief

Where Are You Today?

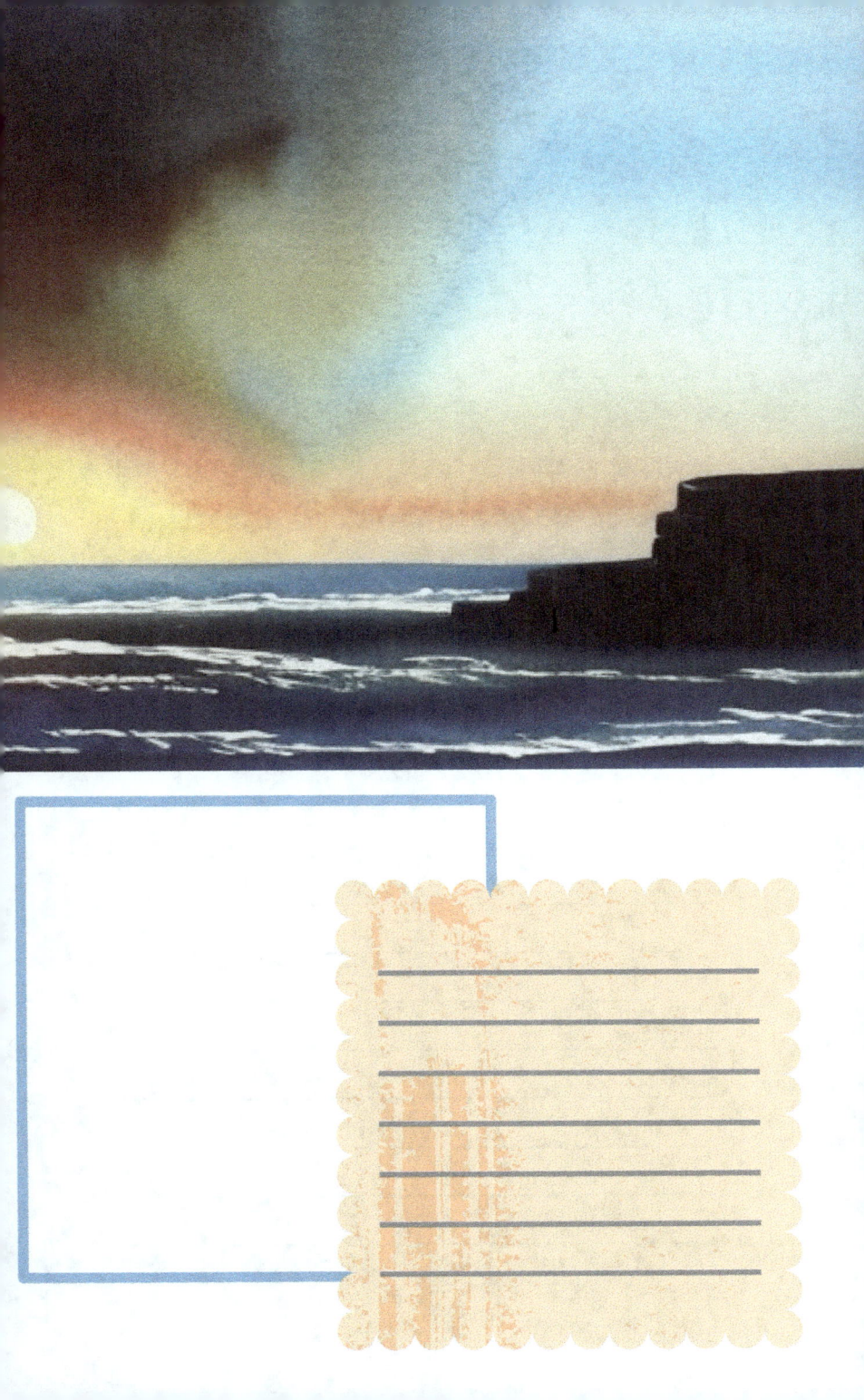

Check-In

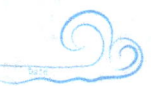

It's a good time to check-in on You. Reflect on your dominant emotions and what's captivating your thoughts? What is your greatest need right now?

_____

_____

_____

_____

_____

_____

_____

_____

_____

_____

_____

Possible Prompts

In what ways are you caring for yourself?

In what ways can you care for yourself better?

What feelings does the idea of processing your grief evoke?

Have you or would you consider grief counseling or attending a support group?

Processing grief may bring forth many tears — but it can also bring joy and laughter. Write about memories that bring you joy.

What are your greatest needs at this moment?

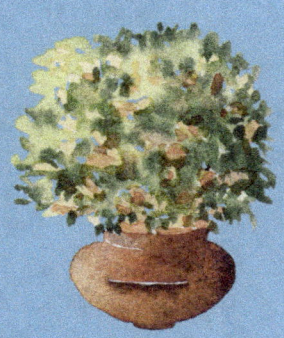

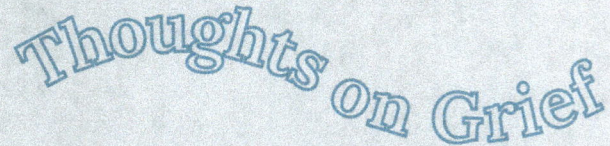

Thoughts on Grief

The best advice I was given was to take it one day at a time.

Put one foot in front of the other and just keep going.

Some days are hard, but get up and get thru that day.

~ Brenda Boling Crossman

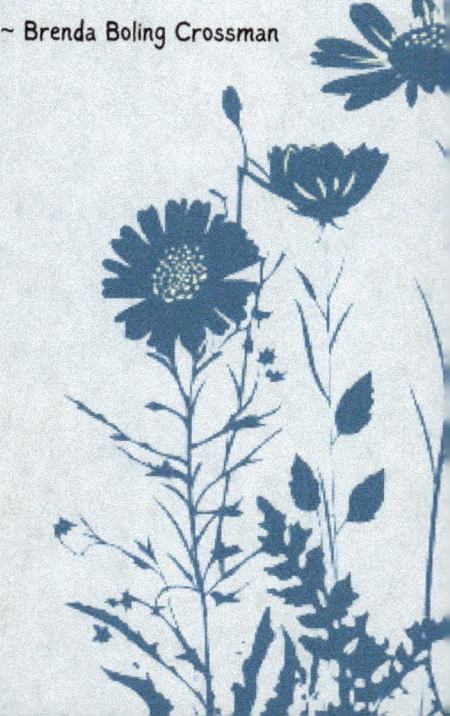

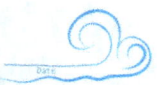

Praise be to the God and Father of our Lord
Jesus Christ, the Father of compassion and
the God of all comfort, who comforts us in
all our troubles, so that we can comfort
those in any trouble with the comfort we
ourselves have received from God.

2 Corinthians 1:3-4

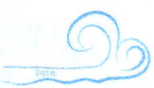

For his anger lasts only a moment, but
his favor lasts a lifetime; weeping may
remain for a night, but rejoicing
comes in the morning.

Psalm 30:5

_____

_____

_____

_____

_____

_____

_____

_____

_____

_____

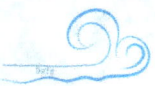

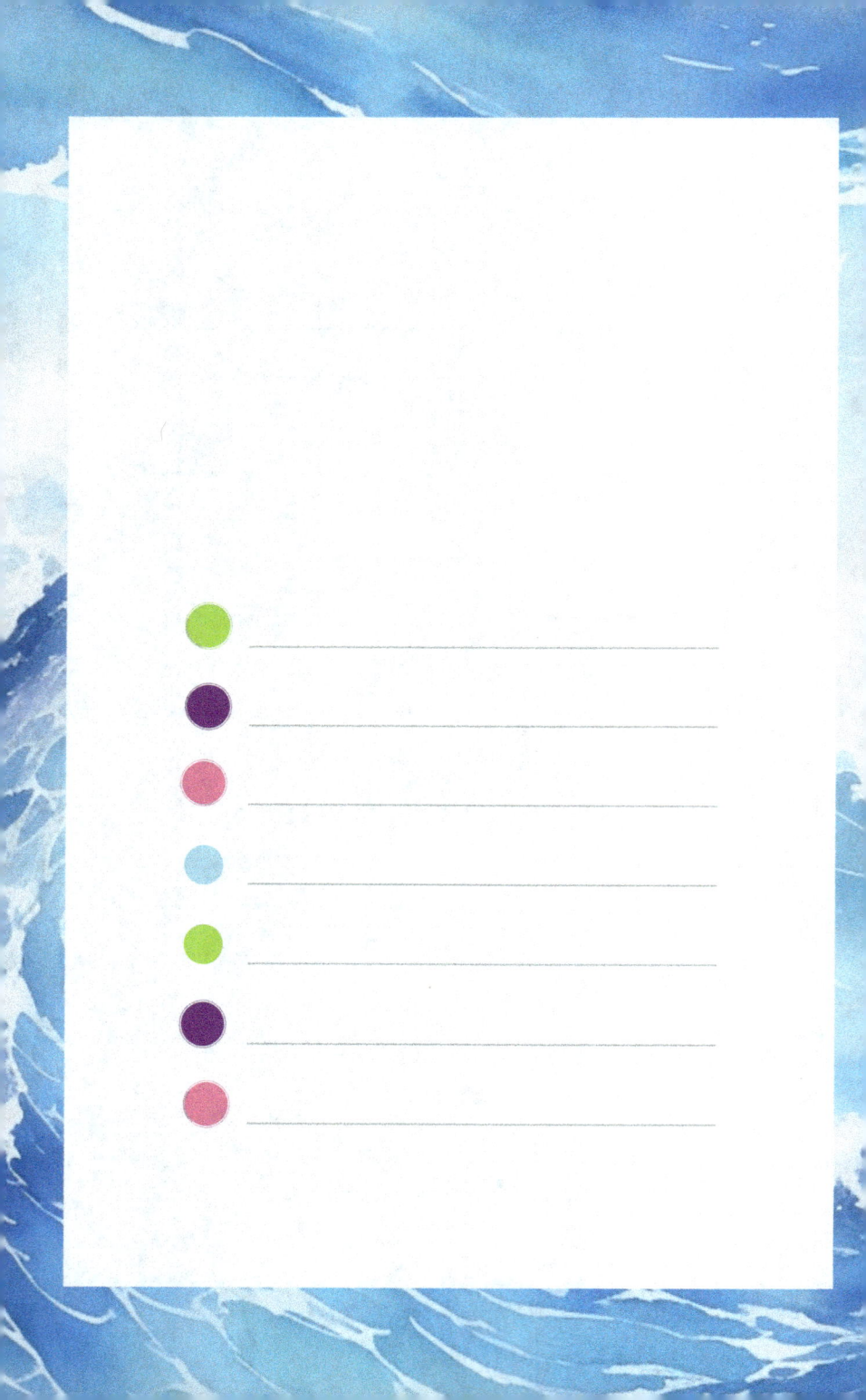

Self-Care Check

Exercise & Activities

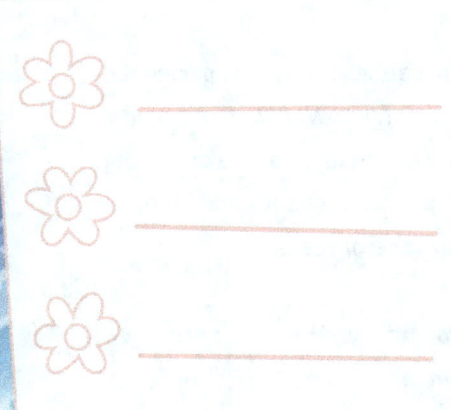

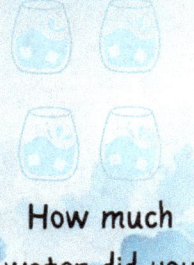

How much
water did you
drink today?

What was the best
part of your day?

Who are you grateful
for? Who or what made
a difference in your day?

It's a Good Time to Read Your Letter

I design journals because I have experienced and witnessed the healing power writing holds; I have marveled at the mind and heart of my past self poured out on a page and I have gleaned wisdom from the process.

You were coached to write a letter to yourself early on in the book. It's time to read it (if you can, out loud ... even better, ask someone in your inner circle to read it to you).

This is an opportunity to celebrate You. Be encouraged with your growth. Open your heart wide enough to fully see the ways in which You are different. Note your growth, healing, and wisdom acquired thus far on your journey.

And my God will meet all your needs according to the riches of his glory in Christ Jesus.

Philippians 4:19

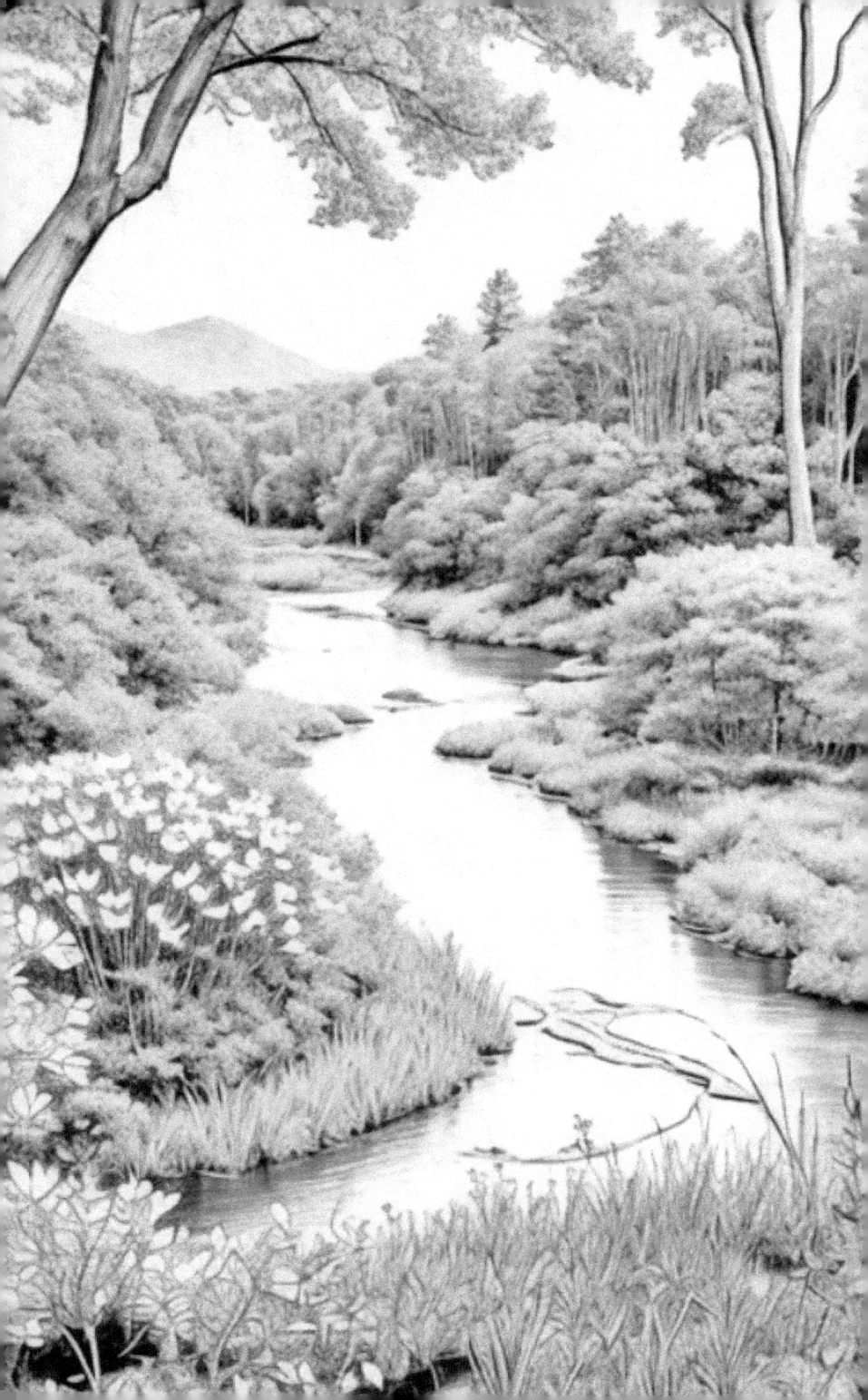

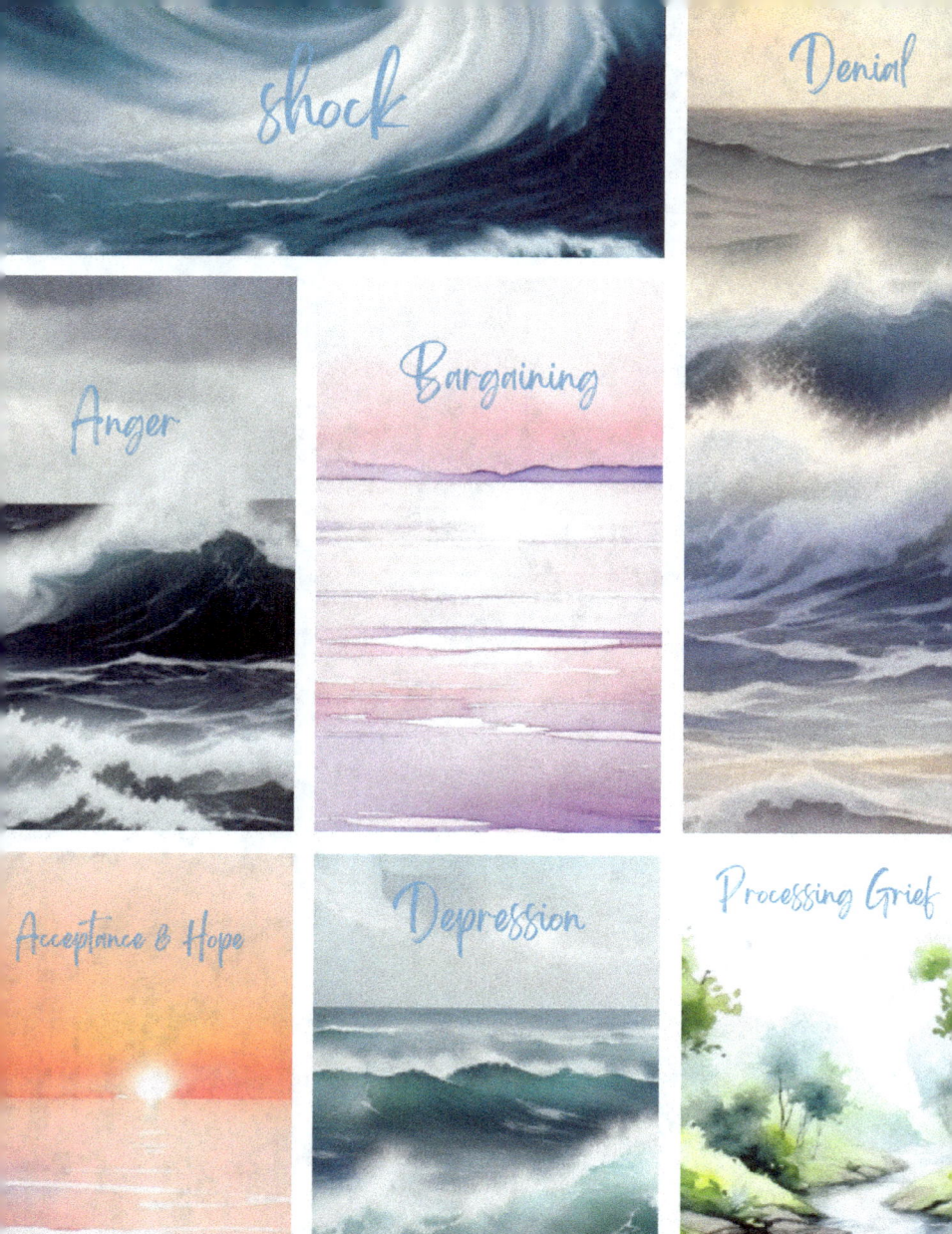

Shock

Denial

Anger

Bargaining

Acceptance & Hope

Depression

Processing Grief

Where Are You Today?

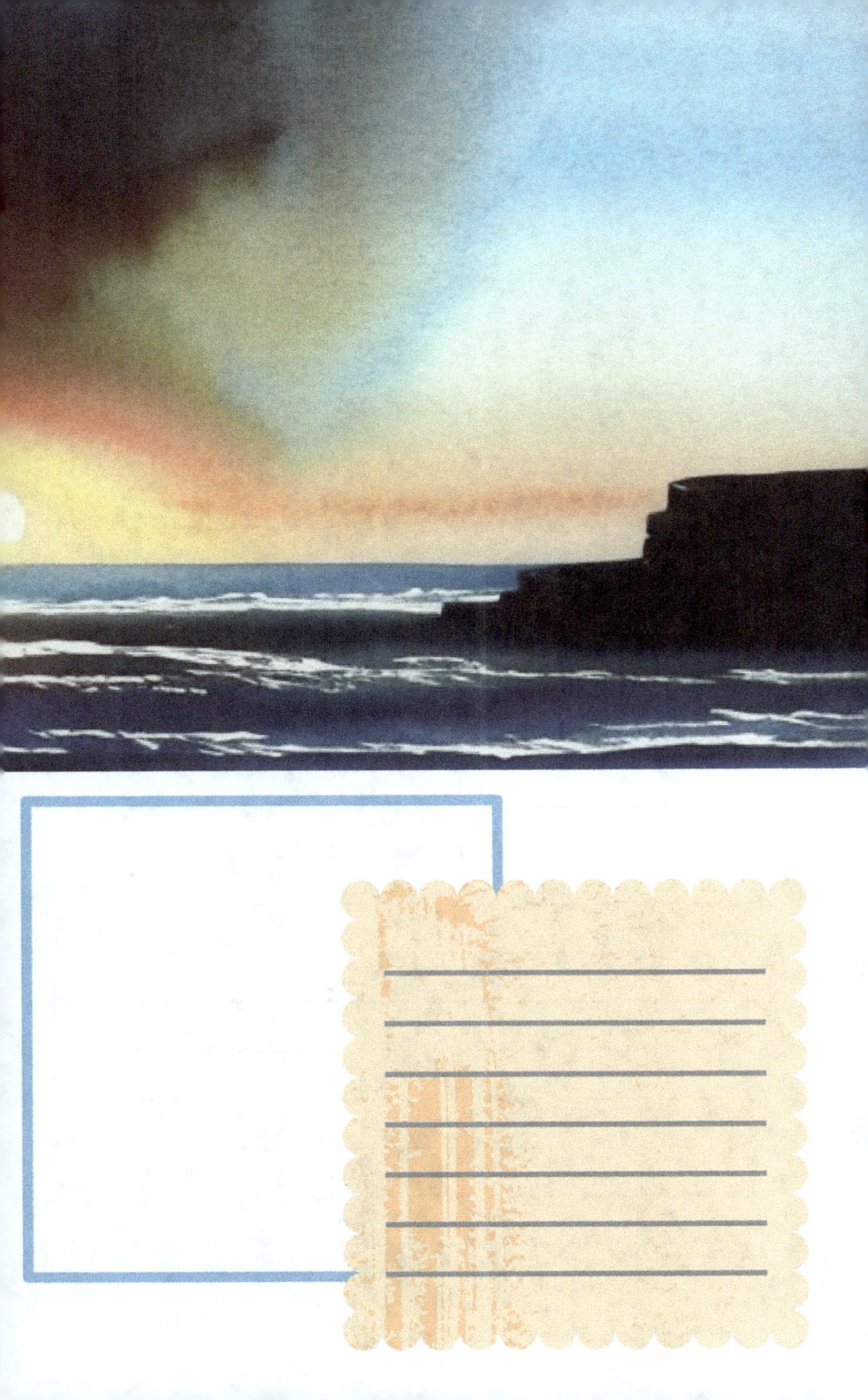

Check-In

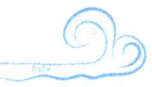

Final Reminder to Be where you Are. Reflect on your dominant emotions and what's captivating your mind? What is your greatest need right now?

_____

_____

_____

_____

_____

_____

_____

_____

_____

_____

Thoughts on Grief

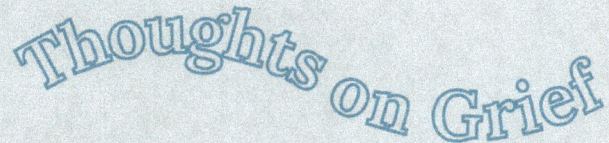

"GET UP, LOOK UP AND NEVER GIVE UP."

Reflect on the wonderful
memories, cry when you need
to, and feel proud to HONOR
the one you love... they are
FOREVER YOURS - a
Guardian angel,
ALWAYS WATCHING FROM
ABOVE!

Wendelin Weaver-Carter

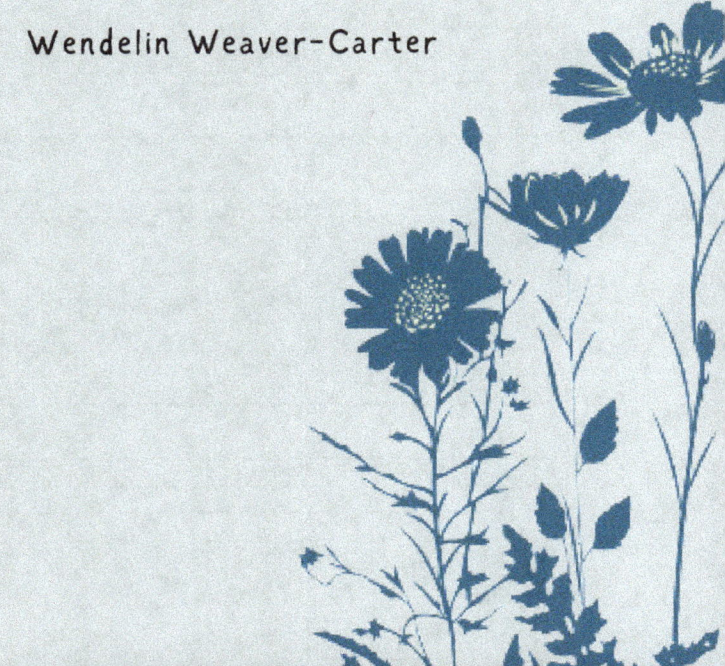

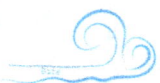

Precious in the sight of the LORD is
the death of his saints

Psalm 116:15

_____

_____

_____

_____

_____

_____

_____

_____

_____

_____

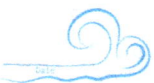

... to proclaim the year of the LORD's favor and the day of vengeance of our God, to comfort all who mourn, 3 and provide for those who grieve in Zion- to bestow on them a crown of beauty instead of ashes, the oil of gladness instead of mourning, and a garment of praise instead of a spirit of despair. They will be called oaks of righteousness, a planting of the LORD for the display of his splendor.

Isaiah 61:2-3

_____

_____

_____

_____

_____

_____

_____

_____

_____

_____

Self-Care Check

Exercise & Activities

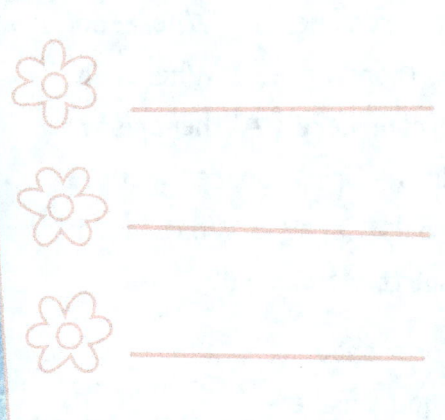

How much
water did you
drink today?

What was the best
part of your day?

Who are you grateful
for? Who or what made
a difference in your day?

Next Steps

Thoughtfully consider your next steps — where will you go from here? Where do you Want to go from here? Where do you Need to go from here? A therapist? A vacation? Join a Grief Share group? Make time for Self-Care? What does your heart and spirit most need?

No one can or should answer this for you. Take a moment to flip through your workbook and read your entries. Deep down, you know exactly what you most need as you are the interpreter of the language of your heart. Listen to what it has to say.

Do not be anxious about anything, but in every situation, by prayer and petition, with thanksgiving, present your requests to God. And the peace of God, which transcends all understanding, will guard your hearts and your minds in Christ Jesus.

Philippians 4:5-7

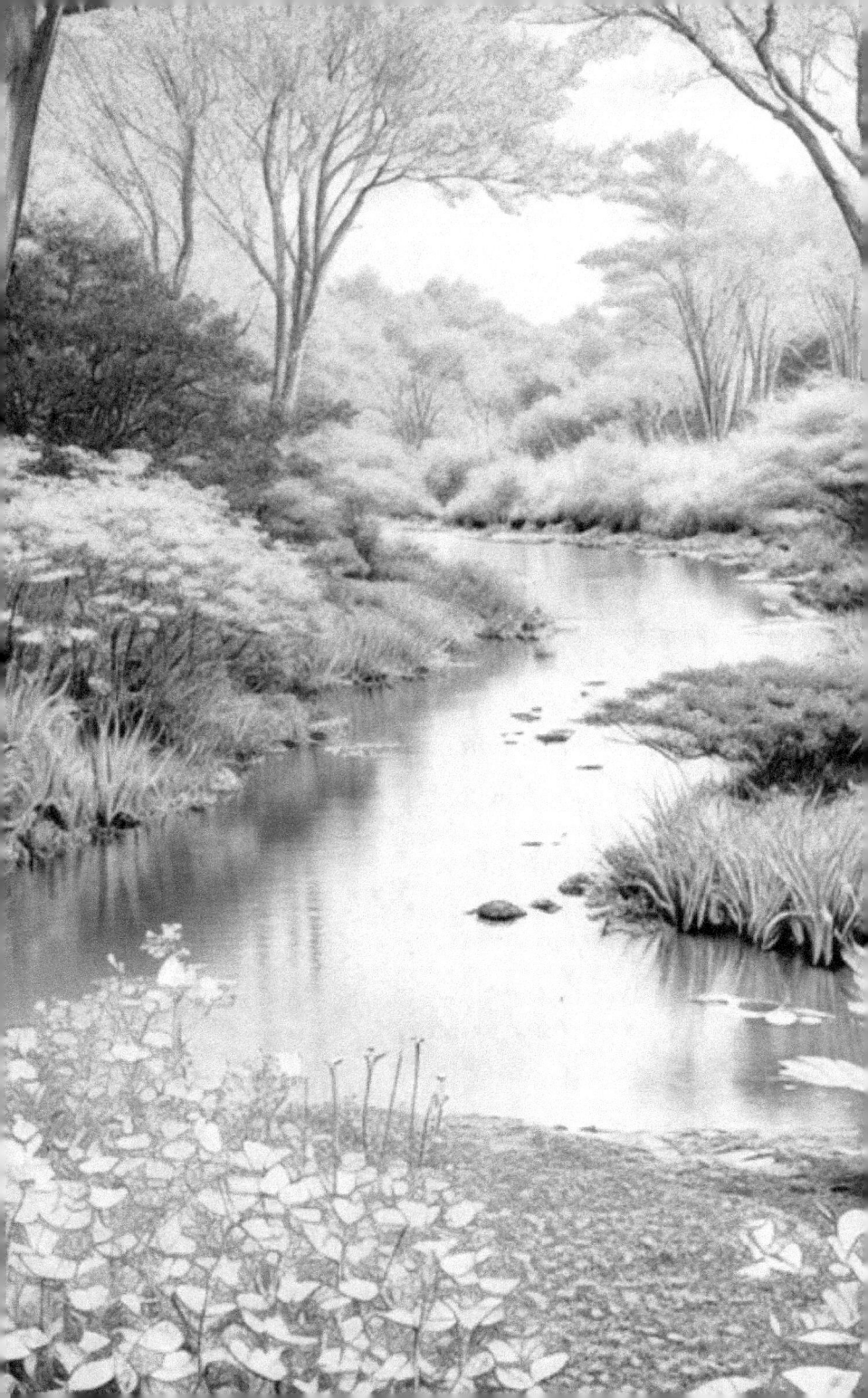

Thoughts on Grief

My best suggestion for dealing with loss is therapy.

I have dealt with a lot of loss in my lifetime and the greatest recommendation I have is to be gentle with yourself and grieve at your own pace.

- don't compare your insides to somebody else's outside... if you don't feel every feeling you're supposed to feel, you'll never fully move on.

-don't be afraid to revisit grief because we all have moments out of the blue that we just need to get out of our system.

~ Anonymous

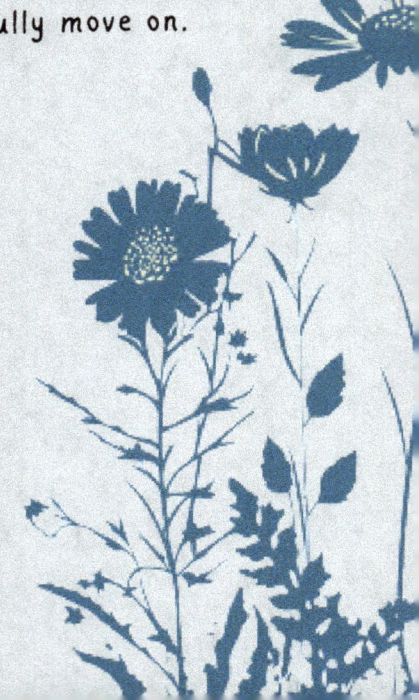

Special Thanks
to our
Featured Contributors

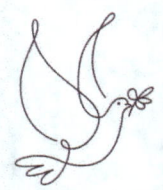

(in alphabetical order by first name)

Angela Miller

Brenda Boling Crossman

David Sherron

Karen Smith

Malika King

Marissa Gilson

Michelle Nelson Kuzma

Nicola Dalbenzio

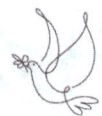

Omar Zaheer

Tonya Vann

Wendelin Weaver-Carter

Praise be to the God and Father of
our Lord Jesus Christ, the Father of compassion and the
God of all comfort, who comforts us in all our troubles, so
that we can comfort those in any trouble with the
comfort we ourselves have received from God.
For just as the sufferings of Christ flow over into our
lives, so also through Christ our comfort overflows.

2 Corinthians 3:1-5

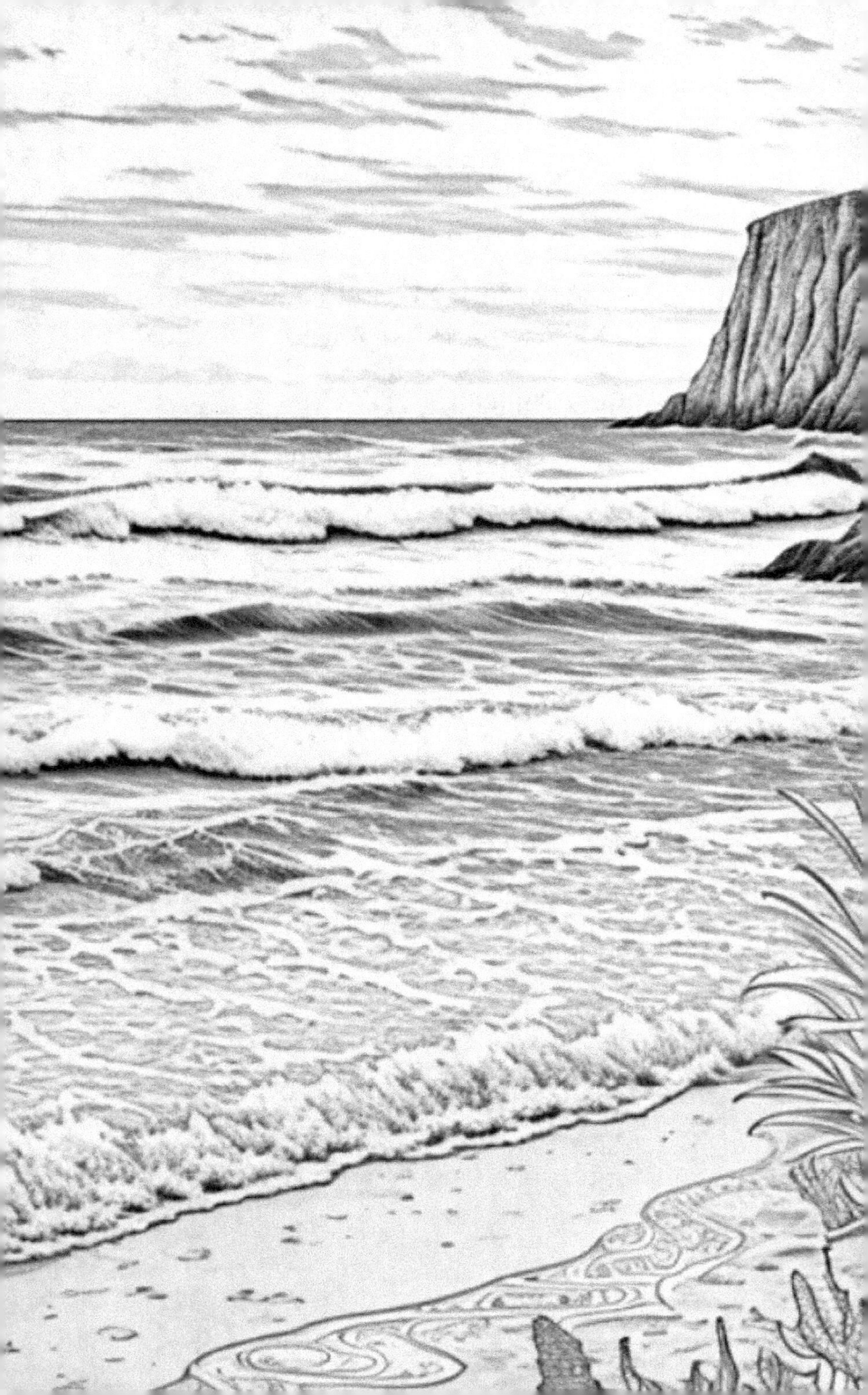

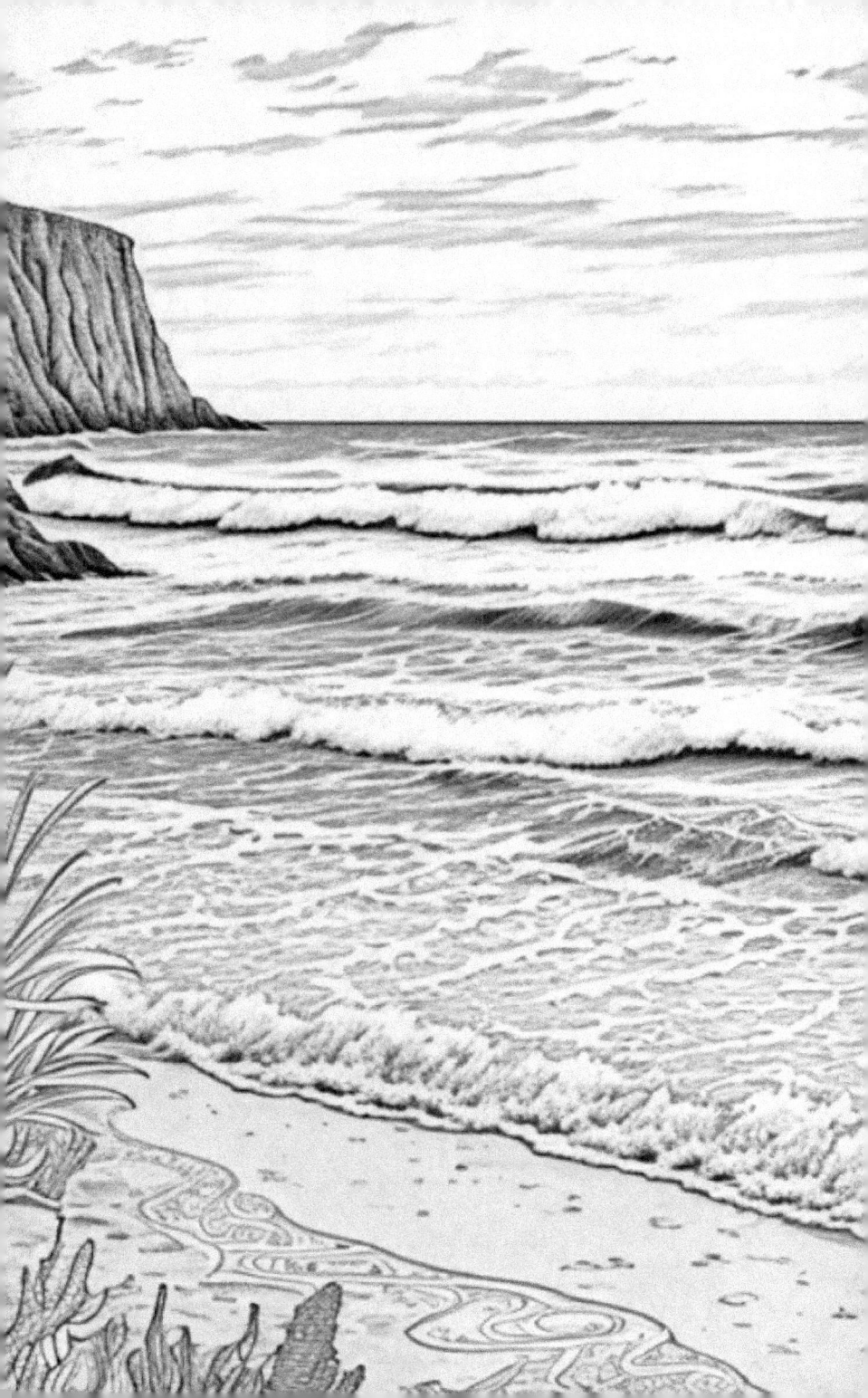